Sirtfood Diet:

2 Books in 1:

Complete Guide To Burn Fat Activating Your "Skinny Gene" + 135 Tasty Recipes Cookbook For Quick and Easy Meals.

|2021 Edition|

© Copyright 2021 by Lola Brown

© Copyright 2021 by Lola Brown

All rights reserved. No part of this guide may be reproduced in any form without permission in writing from the publisher except in the case of brief quotations embodied in critical articles or reviews.

Legal & Disclaimer

The information contained in this book and its contents is not designed to replace or take the place of any form of medical or professional advice; and is not meant to replace the need for independent medical, financial, legal or other professional advice or services, as may be required. The content and information in this book have been provided for educational and entertainment purposes only.

The content and information contained in this book has been compiled from sources deemed reliable, and it is accurate to the best of the Author's knowledge, information and belief. However, the Author cannot guarantee its accuracy and validity and cannot be held liable for any errors and/or omissions. Further, changes are periodically made to this book as and when needed. Where appropriate and/or necessary, you must consult a professional (including but not limited to your doctor, attorney, financial advisor or such other professional advisor) before using any of the suggested remedies, techniques, or information in this book.

Upon using the contents and information contained in this book, you agree to hold harmless the Author from and against any damages, costs, and expenses, including any legal fees potentially resulting from the application of any of the information provided by this book. This disclaimer applies to any loss, damages or injury caused by the use and application, whether directly or indirectly, of any advice or information presented, whether for breach of contract, tort, negligence, personal injury, criminal intent, or under any other cause of action.

You agree to accept all risks of using the information presented inside this book.

You agree that by continuing to read this book, where appropriate and/or necessary, you shall consult a professional (including but not limited to your doctor, attorney, or financial advisor or such other advisor as needed) before using any of the suggested remedies, techniques, or information in this book.

Table Of Contents

WHAT IS A SIRT FOOD?..1

WHAT EXACTLY ARE SIRTUINS?...2

HOW DOES THE SIRTUIN DIET ACTUALLY WORK? 2

WHAT CAN YOU EAT IN THE SIRTFOOD DIET? 3

THE PHASES OF THE SIRTFOOD DIET..3

PHASE 1 3

PHASE 2 3

Safety and side effects...4

THE STEPS OF THE SIRTFOOD MEAL PLAN AND THE 5 DAYS REHEARSAL (PERSONAL EXPERIENCE)
....5

Sirtfood Diet Week 1 / DAY 1 / MONDAY (3 juices, 1 meal) 5

DAY 2 / TUESDAY (3 juices, 1 meal)...5

DAY 3 / WEDNESDAY (3 juices, 1 meal)..5

DAY 4 / THURSDAY (2 juices, 2 meals) 6

DAY 5 / FRIDAY (2 juices, 2 meals) 6

MEAL PLANNING 7

FASTING AND EXERCISE 8

How sirtfoods help us 9

What doesn't kill you makes you stronger 9

And the reason for that is simple...9

And guess what?...10

Everything you need to know 11

TOP TIPS FOR SIRT DIET SUCCESS...13

THE SIRTFOOD RECOMMENDATIONS 15

CAN THE SIRTFOOD DIET BE COMBINED? 17

SHOPPING - WHAT DO I NEED TO GET STARTED?..17

PHASE 1: (DAY 1 - 3) 20

GREEN TEA AND GRILLED CHICKEN KEBABS WITH ROCKET SALAD + CHICKPEAS.....................22

PRAWN ARRABBIATA WITH BUCKWHEAT NOODLES 23

MISO MARINATED TURKEY SCHNITZEL WITH CHILI SALSA AND BUCKWHEAT 24

SIRT MOULES MARINIÈRE 25

SALMON WITH TURMERIC SPICY CELERY 26

ROASTED PORK TENDERLOIN WITH KALE AND WALNUTS 27

SPICED CHICKPEAS WITH BUTTERNUT SQUASH, DATESAND WALNUTS 29

KALE, COCONUT AND TOFU THAI CURRY 30

FRIED NOODLES WITH CHILI AND MISO 31

BRAISED PUY LENTILS WITH KALEAND SLOWLY ROASTED CHERRY TOMATOES.......................32

GREEN TEA TOFU KEBAB WITH ROCKET AND SEAWEED SALAD 33

PHASE 1: (DAY 4 - 7) 34

DATE WALNUT BUCKWHEAT PORRIDGE WITH STRAWBERRIES 35

SIRT SHAKSHUKA (BAKED EGGS WITH SPICY TOMATO SAUCE AND KALE)........................36

OMELETTE WITH ROCKET AND SMOKED SALMON 37

CHICKEN, AVOCADO, ARUGULA AND BUCKWHEAT CRACKERS 38

BUCKWHEAT GALLO PINTO 39

CHILLI AND TURMERIC HUMMUS 40

SCRAMBLED EGGS WITH KALE, RED ONIONS AND TOMATOES 41

SMOKED TROUT, CURD CHEESE AND CAPER CRACKERS 42

KALE AND TOASTED WALNUT SOUP 43

SPICY LENTILS VEGETABLE SOUP...44

SIRT CHICKEN SALAD 45

TUNA AND CHICORY BOATS..46

KALE, RED ONION AND CHEESE FRITTATA..47

LEMON HERB SARDINES WITH ROCKET, AVOCADO AND CAPER SALAD 48

BEAN SEAWEED SALAD WITH MISO DRESSING..49

WHITE BEAN SALAD, KALE AND SUN-DRIED TOMATOES......................................50

CHICKEN SKEWERS WITH SATAY SAUCE AND BUCKWHEAT 51

BAKED COD WITH KALE, CHICORY AND WHITE BEANS 53

CHICORY MADE FROM TOFU AND CHILI WITH ARUGULA WALNUT SALAD 54

ASIAN MARINATED TOFU WITH SATAY SAUCE AND BUCKWHEAT WITH ARAME....................55

TUNA NOODLES...56

FRIED THAI PRAWNS...57

GRILLED TURKEY SCHNITZEL WITH WALNUT, HERB AND CHEDDAR CRUST.....................58

LAMB DATE KOFTA WITH TZATZIKI, ROCKET AND CHILI BUCKWHEAT.................................59

BEEF BURGER WITH SWEET POTATO FRIES 60

SALMON TARTARE WITH ROCKET SALAD 61

STUFFED PORTOBELLO MUSHROOM WITH BRAISED CELERY 62

ARAME AND MISO MEATBALLS WITH CRISPY GINGER KALE 63

PHASE 2..64

What is the magic formula for success? 64

BREAKFAST..65

Sirt cereal 65

Sirt breakfast bar 66

Sirt cocoa pops 67

Sirt fruit bowl..68

Grilled sausages with fried Onions and scrambled eggs with herbs 69

Smoked salmon, arugula and Capers on buckwheat crackers 70

Baked Kipper with Kale and poached eggs...71

Poached egg with rocket, Asparagus and bacon 72

Black currants and oat yogurt 73

Green omelette 73

Choc Chip Muesli 74

Raspberry currant jelly..75

Apple pancakes with Currant compote 75

MEALS...76

Sirt smoked mackerel pie with celery sticks...77

Tuna Niçoise salad 78

Buckwheat pasta salad with artichokes, Parmesan and Parma ham 79

Chicken, Quinoa and Avocado Salad 80

15 minutes Watercress soup 81

Broccoli beans Artichoke salad 82

Smoked trout, watercress and potato salad 83

Sirt green bean salad 84

SNACKS 85

Sirtfood bites 85

Roasted Cajun Nuts 86

Buckwheat and seed crackers 87

Sea salt and apple cider vinegar Popcorn 88

Walnut butter 89

Sirt"Ants on a tree trunk" 89

Peanut energy bar 90

Roasted turmeric nuts 90

Crispy kale seaweed 91

Wasabi peas 92

Fried chili tofu 93

Olive tapenade 94

Crispy fried olives 94

Turmeric apple chips 95

Chocolate treat 95

Frozen chocolate grapes 96

Chocolate Matcha Energy balls 97

DINNER 98

Beef bourguignon with Mashed potatoes and kale 98

Turkish fajitas 100

Sirt Chicken Korma 102

Prawns, Pak Choi and broccoli 103

Cocoa spaghetti Bolognese 104

Baked salmon with Watercress sauce and Potatoes 105

Coq au vin with potatoes and green beans 106

Salmon buckwheat Pasta 107

Cauliflower Kale curry 108

Kidney bean burritos 109

China pan with broccoli, seaweed and Pak Choi 110

Tofu and pumpkin casserole 112

Simple chickpea curry 112

Lentil kale moussaka 114

DESERTS 115

Vegan vanilla Lemon cheesecake 116

Date and mocha cups 117

Chocolate popcorn cake 118

Sirt date pudding with toffee sauce 119

Buckwheat Chocolate chip cookies 120

Quick strawberry mousse 121

Strawberries with Chocolateglaze 121

Hot chocolate pots 122

BEVERAGES 123

Pak Choi and Rucola green juice 123

Watercress and lime green juice 124

Carrot apple Ginger smoothie 124

Berries bananas Smoothie 125

Green tea and Rocket smoothie 126

Chocolate strawberry milk 126

Pineapple Lassi 127

Strawberry Lassi 127

Sirt shot 128

Chili chocolate 128

Hot turmeric milk 129

Vegan mocha milk 129

DRESSING RECIPE 130

Arugula capers salad dressing 130

Chili turmeric salad dressing 130

JUICES & DRINKS 131

Green juice 131

Summer watermelon juice 131

Grape and melon juice 132

SIRT fruit salad 132

Kale currants Smoothie 133

Blueberry smoothie 134

Grasshopper smoothie 134

Power punch Smoothie 135

Date protein smoothie 135

Classic sirt juice 136

Go green smoothie 136

Juicy smoothie 137

QUICK AND EASY 138

Spicy bean burgers with spinach salad..138

Greek salad skewers 139

Florentin eggs 139

Roast Chicken and Pesto Wrap 141

Falafel lunch box...142

Mexican salsa with cheese and cucumber pittas...144

Brie and grape salad lunch box 145

Classic chicken lunch box..145

Turkey escalope with sage, capers and parsley as well Cauliflower couscous 146

Vietnamese turmeric Fish with herbs & mango sauce.....................................147

SALADS..149

French lamb's lettuce 150

Garlic Butter Chicken Arugula salad 150

Edamame salad with grilled tofu 152

Baked salmon salad with creamy mint dressing...153

Pomegranate Feta Walnut Salad...154

Serrano ham salad 155

Potato salad...156

Salad nicoise...156

Sesame Chicken Salad 158

Go-Green Salad...159

Hot chipolata and Currant salad 160

Brie and grape salad with honey dressing...161

Roast Chicken Kale Salad with peanut dressing 162

Smoked trout salad...163

SOUPS ...164

Miso soup ... 164

Mexican chicken soup ... 165

Thai spinach soup ... 166

Savoy cabbage and bacon soup ... 167

Edamame beans Pesto soup ... 168

Spicy butternut squash and kale soup ... 169

Kale Stilton Soup ... 170

Curry broth ... 171

FAST MEALS ...172

Grilled chicken with Lemon and olives ... 172

Delicious salmon and potato Delicacies ... 173

Turmeric prawns ... 174

Vegetables with black Bean sauce ... 175

Beef and broccoli ... 176

Salmon with soy glaze ... 177

Tandoori spears ... 178

Fresh Saag Paneer ... 179

Fragrant Asian Hotpot ... 180

Quick fried beef with salsa verde ... 181

Teriyaki salmon with Chinese vegetables ... 182

Kale tomatoes Pasta ... 183

Curry and rice stew ... 184

What is a sirt food?

What sounds like a treat that comes straight from you.

Science fiction film is a "sirtfood" that is really rich in sirtuin activators. Sirtuins are a type of protein that protects the cells in our body from dying or irritation from health problems.

However, studies have also shown that they can help control your metabolism, build muscle and burn fat. Sirtfoods are all readily available and easily accessible foods.

Some of the best sirtfoods are kale, arugula, parsley, red onions, strawberries, walnuts, extra virgin olive oil, cocoa, curry spices, green tea, and coffee.

Unlike previous popular diet plans that focused on cutting food, with sirtfoods the benefits are achieved through consumption. Along with burning fat, sirtfoods also have the unique ability to naturally satisfy appetite and increase muscle function, making them the best option for healthy weight loss.

Plus, their health benefits are so potent that research studies show they are more effective than prescription drugs at preventing chronic illness, with benefits in diabetes, cardiovascular disease, and Alzhemier to name a few.

So it's no wonder the cultures that eat the most sirtfoods are actually the leanest and healthiest in the world. In the past few years, fasting has actually been the biggest craze, especially the 5: 2 diet, which was the diet-to-do in 2015.

The sirtfood plan is expected to simulate the weight loss results of the fasting diet plan - but without compromising health, fitness, muscle mass or food satisfaction, thanks to new research in this food group.

Just in case 500 calories on Mondays (or even starving all day on Mondays) doesn't really work for you. While it is an effective weight loss routine, the authors are excited to see that it is not just a diet strategy but a well-being and fitness routine.

It doesn't require any calorie restriction or strenuous exercise programs (although staying generally active is obviously an excellent thing. It's neither expensive nor tedious and all of the foods we recommend are widely available. And yes, the list includes dark chocolate (cocoa) and Red wine - so be happy!

It's the year 2020 and already a big favorite and insider tip among the stars.

What exactly are sirtuins?

How sirtuins with NAD + regulate cell health . Imagine the cells of your body like an office. In the office, many people work on various tasks with the aim of remaining profitable and fulfilling the company's mission as efficiently as possible.

In the cells, many parts work on various tasks with the aim of staying healthy and working efficiently for as long as possible. Just as the priorities in the company change due to various internal and external factors, so do the priorities in the cells.

Someone has to run the office and regulate what will be done when, who will do it and when to change course. In the office, that would be your CEO. In the body, at the cellular level, they are your sirtuins. Sirtuins are a family of seven proteins that play roles in cell health.

Sirtuins can only function in the presence of NAD +, nicotinamide adenine dinucleotide, a coenzyme found in all living cells. NAD + is important for cell metabolism and hundreds of other biological processes.

When Sirtuins are the CEO of a company, NAD + is the money that pays the salaries of the CEO and employees while the lights stay on and the office space rent is paid. A company and the body cannot function without them. However, NAD + levels decrease with age, which also limits the function of sirtuins with age. Like all things in the human body, it is not that simple. Sirtuins manage everything that happens in your cells.

How does the sirtuin diet actually work?

Sirtfoods work by activating so-called "lean gene" pathways in the body, the very same genes that are activated when we exercise. This helps the body burn fat in a way that mimics the calorie limit, but without the loss of nutrients or other disadvantages.

A typical weight loss of 3 kg in 7 days was reported by the sample of people who tested the diet, along with increased muscle mass and reports that they felt satisfied and complete with the food intake.

Sirtfoods act as the main regulators of our entire metabolism and above all have an impact on fat loss, while at the same time increasing the muscles and increasing the physical fitness of the cells (this part appealed to me as an enthusiastic athlete)

What can you eat in the sirtfood diet?

As highlighted in the official sirtfood diet, the diet plan program is based on an eating plan that is curated to be full of sirtfoods but lower the total number of calories.

The eating strategy is fairly regulated: for the first three days, dieters are expected to consume just 1,000 calories a day, consisting of a single meal and two green juices. Most of the program encourages dieters to develop meals that are high in sirtfoods (but more on that later) .Some of the staples highlighted in the diet consist of several fruits and vegetables, including kale, strawberries, onions, Parsley, arugula, blueberries and capers. Some grains like buckwheat and walnuts are touted as spices like turmeric. Interestingly, drinks like coffee, matcha green tea, and red and white wine are allowed - as are dark chocolate.

The phases of the sirtfood diet

PHASE 1

The first phase lasts seven days and includes calorie restriction and lots of green juice. It is designed to speed up your weight loss and help you lose 3.2 kg in seven days.

Calorie consumption is limited to 1,000 calories during the first three days of the first phase. You consume 3 green juices per day plus one meal. Each day you can choose from the dishes in the book, all of which include sirtfoods as the main part of the meal. Examples of meals are miso-glazed tofu, the omelette with sirt food or a shrimp pan with buckwheat noodles.

On days 4 to 7 of the first stage, the calorie consumption is increased to 1,500. This consists of two green juices per day and two other sirtfood-rich meals that you can choose from the book.

PHASE 2

Level two takes two weeks. During this "maintenance" phase, you have to keep losing weight. There is no specific calorie limit for this phase. Instead, you consume three meals loaded with sirtfoods and one green juice per day.

Here, too, you can / should select the meals offered in the book. You can repeat these two steps as many times as you think fit and weight loss preference.

Even so, you should remain motivated to "sirtify" your nutritional plan after these phases have been completed by frequently including sirtfoods in your meals.

In addition, you will be asked to keep drinking the green juice every day. With this approach, the sirtfood diet becomes a lifestyle change rather than a one-off diet plan. The sirtfood diet consists of 2 phases.

Stage one lasts **7 days** and combines calorie restriction and green juices. Phase 2 lasts **two weeks** and includes 3 meals and one juice.

Safety and side effects

Although the first phase of the sirtfood diet is very low in calories and nutritionally incomplete, given the short duration of the diet, there are no real safety concerns for the average healthy adult.

For those with diabetes, calorie restrictions and drinking mostly juice for the first few days of the diet can cause dangerous changes in blood sugar levels.

Even so, even a healthy person can experience some side effects - mainly hunger.

If you only eat 1,000 to 1,500 calories a day, almost everyone will be hungry, especially if you consume a lot of juice that is low in fiber.

During the first phase, you may experience other side effects such as fatigue, drowsiness, and irritability due to the calorie restriction.

Serious health consequences are unlikely for the otherwise healthy adult if the diet is followed for only three weeks.

The steps of the sirtfood meal plan and the 5 days rehearsal (personal experience)

Sirtfood Diet Week 1 / DAY 1 / MONDAY (3 juices, 1 meal)

After I actually looked at my brand new juicer and did some shopping, I was finally ready and started to try my hand at it a little. The first 3 days of the sirtfood diet include 3 green juices and only 1 meal, so I knew it was going to be difficult, but actually I was a little amazed. The juices were drinkable and, bizarrely, I felt full all day and didn't feel hungry until around 5 p.m. (which was just an hour before dinner, so completely bearable). The dinner was also very tasty and, above all, filling, but the real highlight of the day were the two pieces of Lindt 85% chocolate that I ate after dinner.

I drank the juices the first around 7.30 a.m. (usual breakfast time), one at 11 a.m. and one at 2.30 p.m. and the chocolate at 9 p.m.

DAY 2 / TUESDAY (3 juices, 1 meal)

The first juice poured over the lips and after the first day of testing continued to taste very good and, above all, was tolerable.

On the other hand, strangely enough, I still didn't feel hungry at all. All day! Not even at 5 p.m. like the day before. And the dinner I chose: "Tandoori Chicken and Peas"

was delicious. In the evening, there was of course a great decadent reward with two squares Lindt 85% and so the second day slowly came to an end.

DAY 3 / WEDNESDAY (3 juices, 1 meal)

I made a few changes to the juice on Wednesday. I spiced up the apple a bit - a whole, not half according to the recipe. After the juices were tolerable for me, I decided to use the same ingredients instead of the 2 juices and to prepare a simple salad. I conjured up a dressing from the salmon juice and ginger as well as from the olive oil. I added it to the kale and then added the rocket, celery, apple and parsley, and a few walnuts. In the end, it made a delicious salad.

DAY 4 / THURSDAY (2 juices, 2 meals)

Thursday began, like all my other days, with a green juice, but this time I knew that only 2 juices had to be drunk and I could treat myself to a delicious meal again around noon and evening. Meal 1 - a remarkably portable strawberry and buckwheat tabbouleh. Dinner was a beef bourguignon with mashed potatoes and kale and it was really delicious.

DAY 5 / FRIDAY (2 juices, 2 meals)

The juice is for breakfast and then the sirt food meals are for lunch and dinner. Lunch was the Sirtfood Supér Salad, a delicious mix of rocket, chicory, avocado, walnuts, capers and a whole host of other sirt foods. The final highlight of the day was dinner: grilled beef with red wine sauce and potatoes.

Meal planning

He really delightful feature of the sirtfood diet is that you have a few weeks to plan your meals. It's something that often costs me half an hour or more on a Monday evening.

Shop

Most of the ingredients are really easy to buy in a regular grocery store: things like kale, celery, parsley, chili peppers, even buckwheat (grits). However, there are some things that are a bit difficult to come by such as coconut flakes, buckwheat noodles - but no problem what the internet is for. Many ingredients are also available on Amazon, such as matcha tea, which also costs a lot. In general, if you're on a tight budget, it can be worth making vegetarian or vegan dishes that focus more on cheap vegetables and staples like beans, lentils and buckwheat and omit or replace some of the more expensive ingredients like buckwheat pasta and matcha Tea.

Juicer

If you're looking to make the juice, there's no getting around it other than buying a juicer, which can be quite expensive. Unfortunately, you can't just blend the ingredients in a blender or food processor. At least I tried when I was preparing for the diet, and in hindsight the consistency wasn't the best and was more like green mud. Therefore, do not necessarily try to save and in this case treat yourself to a juicer that also has enough power.

Beverages

Essentially, you have a choice of water, green tea, black coffee, and black tea (and 2-3 small glasses of red wine in weeks 2 and 3).

Vegan options

Each day has a meat / fish option and a vegetarian / vegan selection. The vegetarian / vegan recipes are easy to prepare and great for hectic days! And they're cheaper too.

Let yourself be inspired

Study participants have lost impressive amounts of weight without losing muscle - sometimes even more likely to gain muscle. Surprisingly, they seldom reported being hungry, a finding that turned out to be unique to sirtfoods' ability to regulate appetite. The average weight loss was 3 kg in seven days after taking muscle gain into account. Inspirational stories had been heard. Ma heard how people got in perfect shape for their wedding day. These results were so successful that these principles were tried on elite athletes, models, and celebrities. The ultimate goal for these test subjects was to improve their body composition and slim down while feeling fantastic. The results that have been achieved have been impressive. After The Sirtfood Diet was published, more and more inspiring success stories about weight loss were received. You've heard of people who lost up to 5 kg in the first week and up to 12 kg in the first month. While this was fantastic in itself, this aspect was even more inspiring.

Fasting and exercise

Two known ways to create positive stress and turn on our sirtuin genes are fasting and exercise. Calorie restriction, a form of fasting that requires a lifetime reduction in calories, has been shown to extend the lifespan of various species.

Exercise is known to have a myriad of health benefits and lower death rates. But as desirable as its sirtuin-activating benefits are, it is not for the faint of heart when it comes to weight loss. The word "hangry" (which, if you haven't already guessed it, is a mix of "hungry" and "angry" representing the bad mood and irritability that results from feeling hungry) is now in the Oxford English Dictionary.

Add in fatigue, muscle wasting, and possibly even malnutrition, and fasting quickly loses its luster. When it comes to exercise, it often takes a heroic effort to be effective for weight loss, as much as we regularly encourage moderate amounts for wellness. You just can't escape a bad diet. If the exertion of fasting or the exertion of heavy physical activity sounds a little too much like hard work, but you want your sirtuin genes to work for you, don't despair, there is a tastier way to be found in food we eat.

How sirtfoods help us ...

Sirtfoods are foods that can mimic the effects of fasting and exercise by activating our sirtuin genes. In this way, we can burn fat, build muscle and promote health. Yes, you got it, you can eat your way to good health and a leaner life! It almost sounds too good to be true, and to really understand how food can do this you need to think very differently about why fruits, vegetables, and plant-based foods are good for you.

So far we've only heard that these foods are good for us primarily because of their content of vitamins, minerals, fiber, and antioxidants. In contrast, we have a completely different point of view and if we're being honest it's one that totally blew us away the first time we ran into it. Plant foods are good for us because they are full of weak toxins. No vitamins. No minerals. No antioxidants.

What doesn't kill you makes you stronger

Natural plant toxins understandably cause stress in our cells, but it's the "good" kind of stress, the kind of stress that gets our sirtuins going and makes our cells adapt and become fitter and healthier. There is a technical name for this phenomenon which is "hormesis". It's an evolutionary survival mechanism, or as we like to say, "What doesn't kill you makes you stronger". Incredibly, all living organisms experience hormesis, including plants. What makes plants special, however, is how devastatingly sophisticated their stress response system is compared to ours.

And the reason for that is simple

Plants are stationary. At first glance this seems really strange, but think about it and you will find that when you are stationary you are at a massive disadvantage. They can't be in search of water, food, shelter, or run from an attacker who wants to make you dinner.

They are literally rooted in place. As a result of this obstacle, plants have developed a dazzlingly highly specified stress response system that helps them adapt to and survive in their environment. It involves making a huge armament of natural plant chemicals to protect them. These plant chemicals are known as polyphenols. When we eat these plants, we not only take in their vitamins and minerals, but we also take in their polyphenols. In fact, we are consuming a number of sophisticated plant stress signals.

And guess what?

Many of these polyphenols have the ability to activate our own innate stress response pathways. We are talking about the exact same stress response pathways activated by fasting and exercise: the sirtuins. Piggybacking on a plant's stress response system like this one is called xenohormesis and it promises to revolutionize our understanding of why certain foods are good for us.

We refer to the foods that are highest in the natural plant substances that activate sirtuins as "sirtfoods".

Farewell, fat!

When people are in this diet, they usually lose weight from both fat and muscle. With the sirtfood diet, however, something completely different has developed. People lost fat without losing muscle. To the great surprise, some people actually built muscle. This is a big deal, no more than losing weight, but rather retaining muscle for a number of reasons because it gives the coveted, toned and lean look.

Even better, holding on to the muscles means reducing the metabolic drop that occurs while losing weight. This muscle continues to burn energy for you even when you are resting. That helps prevent the dreaded weight gain and there are chances in your favor when it comes to permanently reducing weight.

How can this be explained? One of the key members of the sirtuin family, the Sirt-1, hits the fat three times over. First, it blocks the action of something called PPAR-γ, which coordinates the process of making fat in the body.

Second, it increases the activity of PGC-1α, which has the really important job of encouraging our cells to build smaller energy factories that burn fat for fuel.

And to top it off, Sirt-1 causes our fat cells to undergo a personality change, causing them to discard fat instead of storing it.

Muscle building!

That's a hammer blow to the fat, but how do you explain the unexpected effects on the muscles? It turns out that sirtuins also have great effects on muscles. In fact, by activating sirtuins it is not only possible to prevent muscle breakdown, but also to promote its regeneration. This is because Sirt-1 promotes very specialized cells in the muscle - so-called satellite cells - which are responsible for muscle growth and renewal. Indeed, this is the potential benefit to the muscles. Activation of Sirt-1 even appears to be able to prevent the gradual loss of muscle mass and function that occurs with age.

Everything you need to know

What do i need? In terms of equipment, the only essential part of the kit you'll need is a juicer. When it comes to food, most of the ingredients are very familiar and readily available to you. Likewise, for beginners of the sirtfood diet there are some ingredients that we would like to give you a little background knowledge about.

Buckwheat

Buckwheat has recently become the fashionable alternative to cereals, not least due to the success of the sirtfood diet. When it comes to the 100 percent buckwheat puffs and flakes that you'll find in the recipes later on, these are still best sourced from online retailers.

Matcha

Matcha is a concentrated green tea in powder form and what we like to refer to as "green tea on steroids". It is widely available online and is also available in supermarkets. There are two things to consider when buying matcha.
The first is to buy a Japanese version as the alternative Chinese types may be contaminated with heavy metals. The second is to look around for the price. Matcha varies massively in price, with some brands being very expensive, but you can now find good brands at very affordable prices.

Lovage

This previously overlooked herb has been enjoying a renaissance since it was named a top sirt food. If you've never tried it, it tastes like a cross between celery and parsley with hints of curry and aniseed. It's not yet available in supermarkets, but the best place to get it is back online, either as a plant or as a seed.

Chocolate

We have to mention the most popular sirt food: chocolate! It is recommended to use dark chocolate with 85 percent cocoa solids, but it is important to note that even with the same cocoa percentage, not all chocolates are created equal. Some chocolates go through a refinement process called alkalization, which greatly reduces their content of sirtuin-activating nutrients. Since it is impossible to tell from the label which are processed in this way and which are not, I conducted my own research and found that Lindt Excellence 85% cocoa is not alkaline and is the chocolate of choice.

The green juice from Sirtfood

The green juice is an essential part of phase 1 of the sirtfood diet. All ingredients are powerful sirt foods and are contained in every juice. They resemble a strong cocktail of natural ingredients that work together to turn on your sirtuin genes.

All that has been added is a touch of apple for flavor and a little lemon. Don't forget the lemon. Its acidity has been shown to protect, stabilize, and increase absorption of the drink's sirtuin-activating nutrients. It has also been found that fresh ginger really complements the flavors of the juice and brings an invigorating warmth to the mouth.

How to consume your juices

Phase 1, days 1–3: three juices that must be drunk daily. Phase 1, days 4–7: two juices that are to be drunk daily. Phase 2: one juice that is to be drunk daily, with the option of the juice to vary (see recipes)

Who is the diet not suitable for?

While most of the recipes in this book are suitable for the whole family, there are a few important caveats. Phase 1 of the diet is not suitable for children, for people who become pregnant or breastfeeding and for people who are underweight (BMI less than 18.5).

People with significant health problems, medication use, or other reasons to worry before starting the diet should seek advice from their doctor before starting treatment. Pregnant women should limit their caffeine intake to a maximum of 200 mg per day (a cup of instant coffee usually contains 100 mg of caffeine). You should also avoid matcha altogether and don't exceed four cups of regular green tea a day.

The sirtfood diet program was developed for weight loss and is not suitable for children. Likewise, sirt foods with a remarkable caffeine content (matcha green tea and coffee) should not be given to children. However, this does not mean that children cannot benefit from including the many other top sirtfoods in their diets for their exceptional health benefits and from enjoying the many recipes in this book that are designed for family-friendly meals. Although red wine is a sirt food, due to its alcohol content, it should only be consumed in moderation and completely avoided during pregnancy.

Top Tips for Sirt Diet Success

Use this handy guide to get started with the top tips that are tailored to you.

If you work in an office

A little preparation in the morning pays off. A pre-made tasty lunch is something to really look forward to.
- ✓ Buy some green tea bags for the office so you can refill green tea while you work
- ✓ Don't be tempted by the extra goodies and snacks when you hit the stores.
- ✓ If you need to buy lunch every now and then, go for a healthy green salad with leafy greens and lean protein like chicken or fish.
- ✓ On a starting day, buy miso soup (or bring a bottle).

Family life

- ✓ Keep your fridge stocked with blueberries and red grapes: a SIRT booster for you and a healthy snack for your kids.
- ✓ Always cook with olive oil whenever possible, and include onions and green vegetables in family dinners as often as possible.

- ✓ If you're having trouble getting your kids to eat salads, make a large salad with lots of SIRT-rich green leaves and an olive oil dressing.
- ✓ The kids can choose the pieces they eat and you get all of your lovely

SIRTs.

- ✓ Be firm and never allow yourself to eat your children's crusts or leftovers.
- ✓ Buy individual packs of cookies or treats for your kids instead of a tempting family-sized pack. Then buy a 70% / 85% candy bar and keep it just for you.

If you are single

- ✓ Make a load of SIRT-rich meals, refrigerate one or two, and freeze the others. That way, a simple SIRT meal is always waiting for you.
- ✓ Save your red wine when you go out and not drinking at home.
- ✓ Keep a secret stash of dark chocolate handy for emergencies.
- ✓ A stash of prepared kale, spinach, or rocket is great to have on hand at all times. Add them to any meal for an instant SIRT booster.

For vegetarians

- ✓ Eat beans, soybeans, and tofu to increase your protein intake and SIRT levels.
- ✓ Paneer is a great cooked cheese made from skimmed milk that works well in many dishes, not just Indian food.
- ✓ Just remember that combining brown rice and lentils gives you the same essential amino acids that you find in red meat.
- ✓ Peanuts or peanut-based snacks will keep you full, provide SIRTs, and give you extra protein

If you want to get started as a couple

- ✓ Say goodbye to cakes, biscuits and all sorts of sweet treats.
- ✓ Yes, the beer has to be out of the house too.
- ✓ A little competitive spirit should keep you both excited and reduce the chances of you "cheating" on one another.
- ✓ Enjoy a glass of red wine together at the end of a busy day.
- ✓ Consider buying a dark chocolate bar so you don't argue about who ate what.
- ✓ Make a pot of green tea instead of a mug and always make sure there is enough for your partner. You will both end up drinking more tea.

The sirtfood recommendations

Vegetables
- ✓ Artichokes,
- ✓ Asparagus,
- ✓ Bok Choy(Pak Choi),
- ✓ Broccoli Endive,
- ✓ Green Beans,
- ✓ Shallots,
- ✓ Watercress,
- ✓ White Onions,
- ✓ Yellow Chicory

Fruit
- ✓ Apples,
- ✓ black plums,
- ✓ blackberries,
- ✓ black currants,
- ✓ cranberries,
- ✓ goji berries,

- ✓ kumquats raspberries,
- ✓ red grapes

Nuts and seeds
- ✓ Chestnuts,
- ✓ Chia Seeds,
- ✓ Peanut Nuts and Seeds

Grains and pseudo-grains
- ✓ Popping corn,
- ✓ quinoa,
- ✓ whole wheat flour

Beans
- ✓ Broad beans,
- ✓ white beans (e.g. Cannellini or Haricot)

Herbs and spices

- ✓ Chives Dill (fresh and dried),
- ✓ Dried Oregano,
- ✓ Dried Sage,
- ✓ Ginger Peppermint (fresh and dried),
- ✓ Standard Chilies / Peperoni Thyme (fresh and dried)

Beverages

- ✓ Black tea,
- ✓ white tea

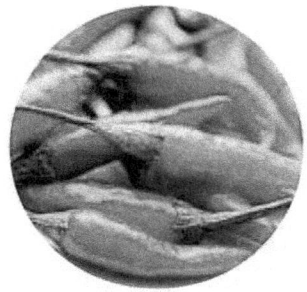
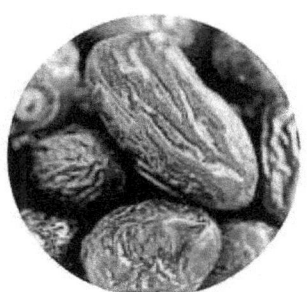

TOP 20 SIRTFOODS
Bird's-eye chilli
Buckwheat
Capers
Celery
Cocoa
Coffee
Extra virgin olive oil
Green tea (especially matcha green tea)
Kale
Lovage
Medjool dates
Parsley
Red chicory
Red onion
Red wine
Rocket
Soy
Strawberries
Turmeric
Walnuts

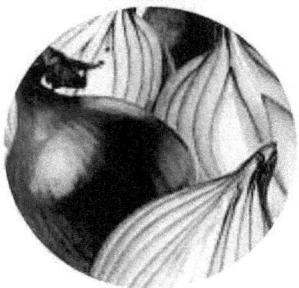
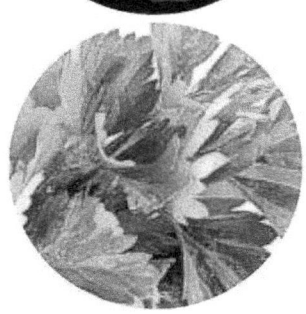
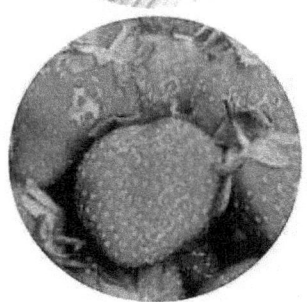

Can the sirtfood diet be combined?

Yes, in any case! In contrast to other diets, the sirtuin diet is perfectly designed to be combined with other diets. With certain diets, the combination has an even better and healthier effect.

These diets include diets such as low carb, paleo, gluten-free or intermittent fasting. Intermittent fasting can be carried out as usual, only that you make sure to consume more sirt foods at meals. When you do that, you have essentially double the effect. When you have an empty stomach, when you are not eating, sirtuin is released, just like when you are eating, because that is where the sirtuin activators in your food take care of it.

Doesn't that sound great? Sirtfoods are also suitable for people who eat gluten-free. Because they are not only low in carbohydrates, but in their natural form do not contain any gluten. You are also welcome to reach out here. Even the low carb food is great for the sirtuin diet. Because almost all top sirt foods are low in carbohydrates, you can incorporate them into your daily meal without any negative consequences. Because plant-based foods are often neglected in low-carb meals, the inclusion of sirt foods has an even better effect. You not only lose weight, but also eat a more balanced and healthier diet!

Shopping - What do I need to get started?

Red grapes

I just can't get enough of it. I make sure that I either eat the delicious SIRTs for breakfast or when I feel like something sweet.

Baby cabbage leaves

Save the large kale for soups and stews, and look for baby kale in the salad aisle. This kale is great for salads or is lightly steamed. It's bursting with SIRTs and is a must-have for any SIRT diet purchase.

Frozen soybeans

I love these beans and highly recommend them to everyone. Cheap and located next to the frozen peas in the supermarket. They are quick to cook and have a wonderful nutty taste. Use them in salads and stir-fries.

70% and 85% dark chocolate

There are different brands with slightly different flavors. As already mentioned, the Lindt brand is a very good address.

Red onions and shallots

In addition to regular white onions for cooking, look for red onions and shallots, which contain even more SIRTs than white onions. Red onions are especially good in salads and keep their shape better than other onions. You can substitute shallots for white onions in pretty much any recipe.

Turmeric, mild chili powder and ground cumin

If you're not used to spices, try this trio with the SIRT-rich turmeric which gives any dish a mild and rich flavor. For two people you will need about ½ teaspoon ground turmeric, 1 teaspoon mild chili powder and ½ teaspoon ground cumin.

Tofu

You can find tofu in the vegetarian aisle in every supermarket. While not your favorite, add it to any dish to boost protein and SIRT levels. Use in any Chinese or seasoned dish, or add to a shrimp dish to increase SIRT levels without adding many calories.

Capers

Adds a salty taste to any sauce or salad. If you add just 1 tablespoon to a dish, you will get an additional 1 tablespoon of SIRT 5 per day. Capers make a delicious and very SIRT-rich salad dressing: 1 tablespoon of capers, juice of ½ lemon, 1 tablespoon of extra virgin olive oil, 1 teaspoon of mustard and lots of salt and pepper.

Light and mild olive oil

When you add mild olive oil as well as regular and extra virgin olive oil to your repertoire, you can use olive oil in both sweet and savory dishes. Mild olive oil does not give a dish the unmistakable olive taste and is also ideal for Asian dishes. Olive oil is so much healthier and more natural than other oils. Olive oil is now my preferred oil in virtually all cooking skills.

"Flavor enhancer"

The food you eat on the SIRT Diet should never be boring. If your dinner isn't satisfying your taste buds, you're much more likely to want to eat something "bad" afterwards. There are many easy ways to do this without increasing the calories. As a bonus, you can sometimes add a few extra SIRTs too.

Salt and freshly ground black pepper

I know it sounds easy, but it makes a huge difference. I don't tend to bring in a lot of salt while I'm cooking, but I always check the seasonings before I serve. If you try a sauce and can't really taste any of its individual flavors, you may have been under-salted. Add a little at a time as over-salted food is even worse. Likewise, I don't think there are many dishes that are not refined with some freshly ground black pepper.

Onions and garlic

If you think about it, onions and garlic are ingredients that you wouldn't want to miss out on in sauces and casseroles. Onions can be cooked slowly for a deep flavor - try sprinkling them with salt to bring out their natural sweetness - or faster for a caramelized golden onion with more bite. Raw red onions add most of the SIRTs then shallot and white onions, and finally garlic. Garlic has a very small amount of SIRTs but adds a lot of flavor and with only 4 calories, you can't go far wrong. Fry for 2 minutes before adding garlic (it takes less time to cook), turn the heat to the lowest setting and place the lid on the pan. In a pan with a lid, onion and garlic can steam and fry, which will keep more SIRTs and cook faster. With the lid closed, cook for 5 minutes to get perfectly cooked onions and garlic.

Parsley

Fresh parsley really enhances every dish. You don't need a lot either, 10 g parsley is enough, which is roughly a small handful. The benefits of adding parsley to a dish are subtle. It doesn't change the taste like some herbs and spices usually do, but it improves it significantly.

Turmeric and other spices

Although turmeric is the only spice that adds SIRTs to a dish, it is fortified when combined with other spices like paprika and cumin.

Phase 1: (Day 1 - 3)

It is a serious kick start to weight loss and good health. This is the so-called "hyper-success" phase and the tried and tested method to lose approx. 3 kg in seven days. The reason it's so successful is because it combines moderate fasting with a diet packed on the rafters of sirtfoods - in short, a powerful two-pronged approach that gets your sirtuin genes going.

Phase 1 only lasts seven days and consists of two different phases. This chapter guides you through the first three days, which are the most intense days.

These consist of: 3 × green sirtfood juices,1 x main meal 15–20 g dark chocolate (85 percent cocoa solids) green juices throughout the day.

For example, you can have a first thing in the morning, a first thing in the morning and a first in the afternoon. To be most effective, they should be taken at least an hour before or two hours after a meal.

Gluten-free, dairy-free, vegetarian, and vegan options are in good hands. I've also included a few quick and easy options for those who are short of time. So, decide on the recipes that are right for you. To save the best until the end, you can eat chocolate from day one. So there are happy days from the start. Most people have their 15–20 g 85% dark chocolate as a mini-dessert after the main meal. In addition to the three green juices, you can also freely consume other liquids in phase 1. The drinks should be calorie-free and preferably contain clear water, black coffee or green tea.

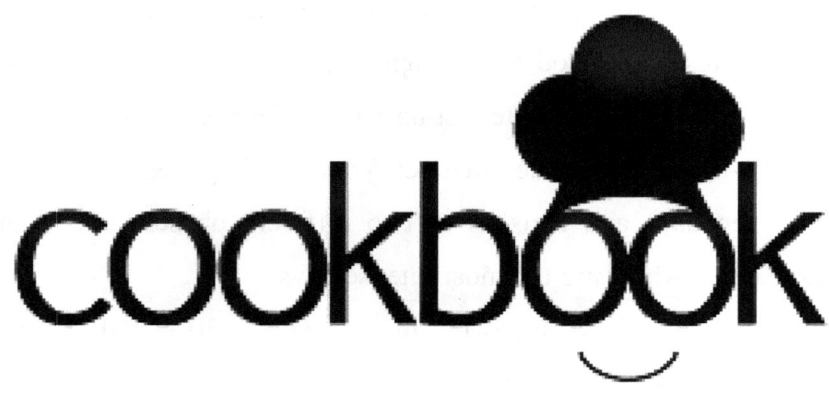

Green tea and grilled chicken kebabs with rocket salad + chickpeas

Preparation time: 15 minutes

Cooking time: 1 hour

Ingredients:

- ✓ 1 medium chicken breast, cut into pieces
- ✓ 60 g red onion, cut into pieces
- ✓ 1 teaspoon matcha
- ✓ 1 teaspoon extra virgin olive oil juice
- ✓ ¼ - ½ lemon, depending on taste
- ✓ 1 clove of garlic(finely chopped)
- ✓ 1 cm fresh ginger, (finely chopped)
- ✓ 1 teaspoon tamari (or soy sauce)

For the salad:

- ✓ 30 g rocket
- ✓ 50 g carrot, grated
- ✓ 40 g celery (finely chopped)
- ✓ 35 g chickpea juice
- ✓ ½ lemon
- ✓ 1 teaspoon tamari (or soy sauce)
- ✓ 1 teaspoon extra virgin olive oil
- ✓ 1 teaspoon sesame seeds
- ✓ 1 cm fresh ginger(very finely grated)

Nutritional values: (1 serving)

Carbohydrates: 12 | Fat: 8 | Protein: 23 | Kcal: 260

Preparation:

- ✓ Mix all kebab ingredients in a bowl and set aside for marinating. The longer you can let the chicken stand, the better - 1 hour would be ideal
- ✓ If you are using wooden skewers, soak them in some water now. Heat your grill on the highest setting. In the meantime, prepare the salad.
- ✓ Mix the rocket, carrot, celery and chickpeas in a bowl. For the dressing mix the lemon juice with the remaining ingredients.
- ✓ Pour the dressing over the salad and mix well. Thread the chicken and red onion on your skewers and grill for 8 to 10 minutes. Then turn them over halfway through cooking. Serve with the salad.

Prawn arrabbiata with buckwheat noodles

Preparation time: 15 minutes

Cooking time: 40 minutes

Ingredients:

- ✓ 65 g buckwheat noodles
- ✓ 1 teaspoon olive oil
- ✓ 125–150 g raw or cooked prawns (ideally king prawns)

For the arrabbiata sauce:

- 40 g red onion, finely chopped
- 1 clove of garlic, finely chopped
- 30 g celery, finely chopped
- 1 chili, finely chopped
- 1 teaspoon herbs of Provence or dried mixed herbs
- 1 teaspoon extra virgin olive oil
- 2 tbsp white wine (optional)
- 1 × 400 g can of chopped tomatoes
- 1 tbsp chopped parsley

Nutritional values: (1 serving)

Carbohydrates: 24 | Fat: 14 | Protein: 11 | Kcal: 310

Preparation:
Make the sauce first

- Fry the onion, garlic, celery, chili and dried herbs in the oil over a medium heat for 1–2 minutes. Turn the heat down to medium, add the wine (if used) and cook for 1 minute.
- Add the tomatoes and let the sauce simmer over medium heat for 20-30 minutes until it's nice, rich consistency.
- If you feel the sauce is getting too thick, just add a little water. While the sauce is cooking, bring a large pan of water to a boil and cook the pasta according to the directions in the package.
- When done, drain, mix with the olive oil and keep in the pan until ready to use. If you are using raw shrimp, add them to the sauce and cook for another 3 to 4 minutes until they have turned pink and opaque.
- Then add the parsley. If you are using cooked prawns, add them with the parsley and bring the sauce to a boil. Add the cooked noodles to the sauce, mix thoroughly but carefully and serve.

Miso marinated turkey schnitzel with chili salsa and buckwheat

Preparation time: 10 minutes

Cooking time: 1 hour 10 minutes

Ingredients:

- 20 g red miso
- 1 teaspoon mirin
- 1 teaspoon extra virgin olive oil
- 125–150 g turkey schnitzel or turkey breast steak
- 1 tbsp ground turmeric
- 50 g buckwheat

For the salsa:

- 130 g tomato
- 10 g red onion
- 1 teaspoon capers
- 1 chili juice
- ½ lemon
- 1 tbsp chopped parsley
- 1 teaspoon extra virgin olive oil

Nutritional values: (1 serving)

Carbohydrates: 32 | Fat: 16 | Protein: 28 | Kcal: 350

Preparation:

- Mix the miso, mirin and olive oil and rub the mixture into the schnitzel. Ideally, you should let this marinate for 1 hour, but if you want to use it right away, you can too.
- Heat your grill on the highest setting. Put 500 ml of water with the turmeric in a saucepan, bring it to a boil and cook the buckwheat as indicated on your package.
- Drain and save. In the meantime, prepare the salsa.
- Finely chop tomatoes, red onions, capers and chili, making sure to keep all of the liquid away from the tomato.
- Mix with lemon juice, parsley and oil. Grill the turkey for 5 minutes on each side, watching carefully so as not to burn the marinade.
- Serve with salsa and buckwheat.

Sirt Moules Marinière

Preparation time: 10 minutes

Cooking time: 30 minutes

Ingredients:

- 300 g live mussels
- 50 g buckwheat
- 30 g kale, roughly chopped
- 40 g red onion, finely chopped
- 40 g celery, finely chopped
- 2 cloves of garlic, finely chopped
- 2 tbsp chopped parsley
- 100 ml white wine
- 1 tbsp extra virgin olive oil

Nutritional values: (1 serving)

Carbohydrates: 15 | Fat: 13 | Protein: 24 | Kcal: 220

Preparation:

✓ To prepare the clams, remove their beards. This is a thread-like membrane that can be easily peeled off.

✓ Gently tap each clam and discard any non-closing clams.

✓ Place the mussels in a colander and wash them under running water to remove any dirt particles. If possible, try to use your mussels on the day of purchase to maximize freshness.

✓ Put 750 ml of water in a saucepan, bring to a boil and cook the buckwheat according to the instructions in the package. Add the kale for the last 5 minutes of cooking time. Drain and set aside. Put a large saucepan with a lid on high heat until it begins to smoke.

✓ Add the cleaned clams. Immediately add the red onion, celery, garlic, parsley and wine.

✓ Mix thoroughly and place a lid on the pan to steam the clams and keep them on high heat. The mussels cook very quickly and should be ready in 2 to 3 minutes. At this point they should all be open.

✓ Stir them about every 30 seconds to regulate the heat in the pan. Be careful not to over-cook them as they will become chewy and tasteless. Stir in the olive oil, buckwheat and kale and serve.

Salmon with turmeric spicy celery

Preparation time: 15 minutes

Cooking time: 25 minutes

Ingredients:

- 1 teaspoon ground turmeric
- 1 teaspoon extra virgin olive oil juice
- ¼ lemon
- 125–150 g peeled salmon fillet

For the spicy celery

- 1 teaspoon extra virgin olive oil
- 40 g red onion, finely chopped
- 1 clove of garlic, finely chopped
- 1 cm fresh ginger, finely chopped
- 1 chili, finely chopped
- 150 g celery, cut into 2 cm pieces
- 1 teaspoon mild curry powder
- 130 g (approx. 1) tomato, cut into 8 pieces
- 100 ml of chicken or vegetable stock
- 60 g tinned and drain green lentils
- 1 tbsp chopped parsley

Nutritional values: (1 serving)

Carbohydrates: 11 | Fat: 23 | Protein: 26 | Kcal: 410

Preparation:

- Heat the oven to 200ºC / gas 6. Start with the spicy celery. Heat a pan over medium-low heat, add the olive oil, then the onion, garlic, ginger, chilies and celery.
- Fry lightly for 2-3 minutes or until soft but not colored, then add the curry powder and cook for another minute.
- Add the tomato, then the broth and lentils and let simmer gently for 10 minutes. Depending on how crispy you like your celery, you can lengthen or shorten the cooking time.
- In the meantime, mix the turmeric, oil and lemon juice and spread over the salmon. Place on a baking sheet and cook for 8-10 minutes.
- Finally stir the parsley through the celery and serve with the salmon.

Roasted pork tenderloin with Kale and walnuts

Preparation time: 10 minutes

Cooking time: 15 minutes

Ingredients:

- 125–150 g pork tenderloin
- 1 teaspoon extra virgin olive oil
- Juice of ¼ lemon
- 1 teaspoon ground turmeric

For the buckwheat

- 1 tbsp ground turmeric
- 50 g buckwheat

For the vegetables

- 1 teaspoon extra virgin olive oil
- 40 g red onion, finely chopped
- 1 clove of garlic, finely chopped
- 1 chili, finely chopped
- 1 cm fresh ginger, finely chopped
- 1 teaspoon ground cumin
- 50 g kale, roughly chopped
- 20 g green beans, halved
- 20 g celery, thinly sliced
- 100 ml of chicken broth
- 1 teaspoon tamari (or soy sauce)
- 20 g chopped walnuts
- 1 tbsp chopped coriander

Nutritional values: (1 serving)

Carbohydrates: 13 | Fat: 31 | Protein: 22 | Kcal: 380

Preparation:

First, make the buckwheat:

- ✓ Put 500 ml of cold water in a saucepan, add the turmeric and bring to a boil. Cook the buckwheat according to the directions in the package and set aside until needed. Cut the fat off the pork and cut it into 1 cm thick slices.
- ✓
- ✓ • Mix with olive oil, lemon juice and turmeric. Heat a pan over medium-

- ✓ high heat, add the pork, and saute for 3 to 4 minutes until cooked through.

- ✓ Then take it out of the pan and place it on the plate. Add the olive oil for the vegetables to the pan over low heat.
- ✓
- ✓ Add the red onion, garlic, chili and ginger. When they are soft but not colored, add the cumin and cook for another minute.
- ✓
- ✓ Add the kale, green beans, and celery and gently cook for 2-3 minutes.
- ✓
- ✓ Then add the broth and tamari. Cook over low to medium heat or until vegetables are tender for a few minutes.

- ✓ Add walnuts, coriander and boiled pork, mix well and serve with the buckwheat.

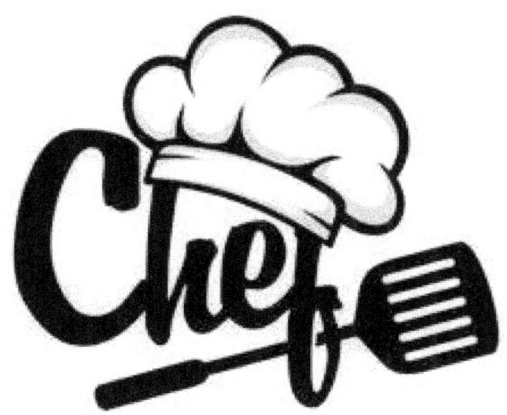

Spiced chickpeas with Butternut squash, datesand walnuts

Preparation time: 15 minutes

Cooking time: 20 minutes

Ingredients:

- ✓ 2 large Medjool dates, pitted and chopped
- ✓ 100 ml of hot vegetable stock
- ✓ 100 g butternut squash
- ✓ 1 teaspoon extra virgin olive oil
- ✓ 40 g red onion, sliced
- ✓ 1 chili, finely chopped
- ✓ 1 clove of garlic, finely chopped
- ✓ 1 teaspoon ground turmeric
- ✓ 1 teaspoon paprika
- ✓ ½ teaspoon ground cinnamon
- ✓ 1 teaspoon ground cumin
- ✓ 150 g canned chickpeas, drained
- ✓ 20 g chopped walnuts
- ✓ 1 tbsp chopped parsley
- ✓ 15 g rocket

Nutritional values: (1 serving)

Carbohydrates: 11 | Fat: 33 | Protein: 24 | Kcal: 390

Preparation:

- ✓ Place the chopped dates in the hot broth and set aside until needed. Peel the butternut squash and cut into bite-sized pieces.
- ✓ Put in a pan with boiling water and simmer for 10 to 15 minutes. Be careful that it doesn't get muddy.
- ✓ Drain and set aside. Heat a saucepan or casserole over low heat, add olive oil, onion, chili and garlic and fry gently for 2 minutes.
- ✓ Add the turmeric, red pepper, cinnamon and cumin and cook for another minute or so.
- ✓ Add the chickpeas, walnuts and the date broth mixture and bring to a boil.
- ✓ Cook for a minute then add the pumpkin and parsley. Just before serving, remove the pan from the heat and stir through the arugula.

Kale, coconut and Tofu Thai Curry

Preparation time: 10 minutes

Cooking time: 30 minutes

Ingredients:

- ✓ 100 ml vegetable broth
- ✓ 1 teaspoon tamari (or soy sauce)
- ✓ 150 ml coconut milk
- ✓ 50 g kale, roughly chopped
- ✓ 30 g carrots, roughly chopped
- ✓ 30 g celery, roughly chopped
- ✓ 150 g firm tofu, cut into 2 cm cubes
- ✓ 6–8 basil leaves

For the curry paste

- ✓ 30 g red onion, roughly chopped
- ✓ 1 cm fresh ginger, roughly chopped
- ✓ 1 clove of garlic, roughly chopped
- ✓ 1 chili, roughly chopped
- ✓ 1 lemongrass stalk, roughly chopped
- ✓ 1 tbsp chopped parsley
- ✓ 1 teaspoon ground turmeric
- ✓ 1 teaspoon ground cumin
- ✓ 1 teaspoon extra virgin olive oil

For the buckwheat

- ✓ 1 tbsp ground turmeric 50g buckwheat

Nutritional values: (1 serving)

Carbohydrates: 8 | Fat: 17 | Protein: 25 | Kcal: 220

Preparation:

- ✓ Put all the ingredients for the paste in a blender and mix until a fine paste is formed.
- ✓ Transfer the paste to a saucepan and gently cook over low heat for 2-3 minutes.
- ✓ Add the stock, tamari and coconut milk and cook for 20 minutes. In the meantime, put 500 ml of cold water in a saucepan, add the turmeric and bring to a boil.
- ✓ Cook the buckwheat according to the instructions in the package and set aside until needed.
- ✓ Add the kale, carrot and celery to the curry and cook for another 10 minutes.
- ✓ Stir in tofu and basil, bring to the boil, remove from heat immediately and serve with the cooked buckwheat.

Fried noodles with Chili and miso

Preparation time: 15 minutes

Cooking time: 15 minutes

Ingredients:

- ✓ 75 g buckwheat noodles
- ✓ 2 teaspoons of extra virgin olive oil
- ✓ 5 grams of dried arame
- ✓ 25 g miso paste
- ✓ 40 g red onion, thinly sliced
- ✓ 40 g celery, thinly sliced
- ✓ 1 clove of garlic, finely chopped
- ✓ 1 cm fresh ginger, finely chopped
- ✓ 1 chili, finely chopped
- ✓ 50 g grated carrots
- ✓ 30 g cut mushrooms
- ✓ 50 g kale, roughly chopped
- ✓ 1 tbsp chopped coriander

Nutritional values: (1 serving)

Carbohydrates: 34 | Fat: 17 | Protein: 15 | Kcal: 360

Preparation:

- ✓ Cook the pasta according to the instructions in the package. When done, drain, mix with 1 teaspoon of olive oil and set aside until needed.
- ✓ Cover the arame with boiling water, let it sit for 5 minutes then drain.
- ✓ Mix 100 ml of boiling water with the miso paste and stir until everything is dissolved. Heat the remaining teaspoon of olive oil in a pan, add onion, celery, garlic, ginger and chili and fry for 1–2 minutes over a medium heat.
- ✓ Add the carrot, mushrooms and kale, raise the heat to medium and cook for 2-3 minutes.
- ✓ Mix in the noodles and continue cooking for about a minute, stirring constantly to keep the noodles from sticking.
- ✓ Add the miso broth, bring to a boil, remove from heat and let stand for 1 minute - the pasta should absorb most of the remaining liquid. Stir in the chopped coriander and serve.

Braised puy lentils with kaleand slowly roasted Cherry tomatoes

Preparation time: 15 minutes

Cooking time: approx. 1 hour

Ingredients:

- ✓ 8 halved cherry tomatoes
- ✓ 2 teaspoons of extra virgin olive oil
- ✓ 40 g red onion, thinly sliced
- ✓ 1 clove of garlic, finely chopped
- ✓ 40 g celery, thinly sliced
- ✓ 40 g carrots, thinly sliced
- ✓ 1 teaspoon paprika
- ✓ 1 teaspoon thyme (dried or fresh)
- ✓ 75 g of dried puy lentils
- ✓ 220 ml vegetable broth
- ✓ 50 g kale, roughly chopped
- ✓ 1 tbsp chopped parsley
- ✓ 20 g rocket

Nutritional values: (1 serving)
Carbohydrates: 27 | Fat: 19 | Protein: 9 | Kcal: 310

Preparation:

- Preheat your oven to 120°C / gas ½. Place the tomatoes in a small roasting tin and roast in the oven for 35–45 minutes.
- Heat a saucepan over low to medium heat. Add 1 teaspoon of olive oil with the red onion, garlic, celery and carrot and fry for 1–2 minutes until soft.
- Stir in paprika and thyme and cook for another minute. Wash the lentils in a fine-mesh colander and add them to the pan with the broth.
- Bring to a boil then reduce the heat and simmer gently on the pan for 20 minutes with a lid.
- Stir the pan about every 7 minutes and add a little water if the level drops too much.
- Add the kale and cook for another 10 minutes. When the lentils are cooked, stir in the parsley and roasted tomatoes.
- Serve with rocket, drizzled with the remaining teaspoon of olive oil.

Green tea tofu kebab with rocket and seaweed salad

Preparation time: 15 minutes

Cooking time: approx. 1 hour

Ingredients:

- ✓ 150 g firm tofu, cut into pieces
- ✓ 60 g red onion, cut into pieces
- ✓ 1 teaspoon matcha green tea
- ✓ 1 teaspoon extra virgin olive oil juice
- ✓ ¼ - ½ lemon depending on your preference
- ✓ 1 clove of garlic, finely chopped
- ✓ 1 cm fresh ginger, finely chopped
- ✓ 1 teaspoon tamari (or soy sauce)

For the salad

- ✓ 7 g arame juice of ½ lime
- ✓ 1 teaspoon tamari (or soy sauce)
- ✓ 1 teaspoon extra virgin olive oil
- ✓ 1 teaspoon sesame 1 cm fresh ginger, finely grated
- ✓ 50 g grated carrot
- ✓ 40 g celery, thinly sliced
- ✓ 40 g rocket

Nutritional values: (1 serving)
Carbohydrates: 23 | Fat: 9 | Protein: 12 | Kcal: 220

Preparation:

- Mix the tofu and red onion with all the remaining ingredients for the kebab. The longer you can marinate the tofu, the better, ideally 1 hour.
- If you are using wooden skewers, soak them in some water now. Heat your grill on the highest setting.
- Put the arame in a bowl and cover with boiling water. Leave on for 5 minutes, then drain and dry thoroughly

For the dressing:

- Mix the lime juice, tamari, olive oil and sesame seeds.
- Grate the ginger into the mixture as finely as possible. Thread the tofu and red onion on your skewers, grill them for 8-10 minutes then turn them halfway through cooking.
- Mix the carrot, celery and arugula for the salad. When your kebabs are ready, toss the dressing through the salad and serve.

Phase 1: (Day 4 - 7)

With the first three days of phase 1, you are well on the way to getting started successfully with sirtfood. In fact, this is the hardest part as you will be increasing your food intake over the next four days.

You do this by leaving out one of the green juices and adding a second meal each day. You can eat up to 1,500 calories per day during the four-day period.

These consist of:
- ✓ 2 × green sirtfood juices
- ✓ 2 × main meals.

When it comes to green juices, it's still good to spread them out throughout the day. We recommend you have one either in the morning or in the morning and afternoon.

As before, they should be taken at least an hour before or two hours after eating.

The good news is you can now enjoy two delicious meals packed with sirtfood every day. The most common way to do this is to have the first meal during the day and the second with dinner in the evening.

However, be flexible and adapt them to what works for you. The meal of the day can be taken for breakfast, brunch, or lunch, whatever works for you.

Date walnut buckwheat porridge with strawberries

Preparation time: 10 minutes

Cooking time: -

Ingredients:

- ✓ 200 ml milk or dairy-free alternative
- ✓ 1 chopped Medjool date
- ✓ 35 g buckwheat flakes
- ✓ 1 teaspoon walnut butter or 4 chopped walnut halves
- ✓ 50 g peeled strawberries

Nutritional values: (1 serving)

Carbohydrates: 25 | Fat: 5 | Protein: 5 | Kcal: 170

Preparation:

- ✓ Put the milk and date in a pan, heat slightly, then add the buckwheat flakes and cook until the porridge has the desired consistency.
- ✓ Stir in the walnut butter or walnuts, cover with the strawberries and
- ✓ serve.

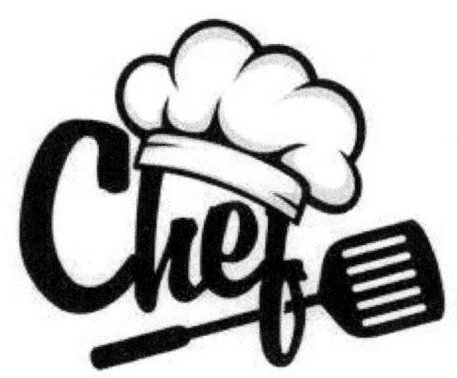

Sirt Shakshuka (baked eggs with spicy Tomato sauce and kale)

Preparation time: 10 minutes

Cooking time: 40 minutes

Ingredients:

- ✓ 1 teaspoon extra virgin olive oil
- ✓ 40 g red onion, finely chopped
- ✓ 1 clove of garlic, finely chopped
- ✓ 30 g celery, finely chopped
- ✓ 1 chili, finely chopped
- ✓ 1 teaspoon ground cumin
- ✓ 1 teaspoon ground turmeric
- ✓ 1 teaspoon paprika
- ✓ 1 × 400 g can of chopped tomatoes
- ✓ 30 g kale, stalks removed, roughly chopped
- ✓ 1 tbsp chopped parsley
- ✓ 2 medium-sized eggs

Nutritional values: (1 serving)
Carbohydrates: 8 | Fat: 11 | Protein: 25 | Kcal: 180

Preparation:

- Heat a small, deep pan over medium-low heat. Add the oil and sauté onion, garlic, celery, chili and spices for 1–2 minutes.
- Add the tomatoes and let the sauce simmer gently for 20 minutes, stirring occasionally.
- Add the kale and cook for another 5 minutes. If you feel the sauce is getting too thick, just add a little water.
- When your sauce has a nice, rich consistency, stir in the parsley. Make two small indentations in the sauce and crack each egg in it.
- Reduce the heat to the lowest setting and cover the pan with a lid or foil.
- Let the eggs boil for 10–12 minutes. At this point, the whites should be firm while the yolks are still runny.
- Cook for another 3–4 minutes if you want the yolks to be firm. Serve immediately - ideally straight from the pan.

Omelette with rocket and smoked salmon

Preparation time: 5 minutes

Cooking time: 10 minutes

Ingredients:

- ✓ 2 medium-sized eggs
- ✓ 100 g smoked salmon, sliced
- ✓ ½ teaspoon capers
- ✓ 10 g chopped rocket
- ✓ 1 teaspoon chopped parsley
- ✓ 1 teaspoon extra virgin olive oil

Nutritional values: (1 serving)

Carbohydrates: 6 | Fat: 13 | Protein: 21 | Kcal: 150

Preparation:

- ✓ Put the eggs in a bowl and whisk well. Add the salmon, capers, arugula and parsley.
- ✓
- ✓ Let the olive oil get hot in a non-stick pan. Add the egg mixture and use a spatula or fish slice to stir the mixture in the pan until it is even.
- ✓
- ✓ Reduce the heat and let the omelette cook through. Slide the spatula around the edges and roll or fold the omelette in half for serving.

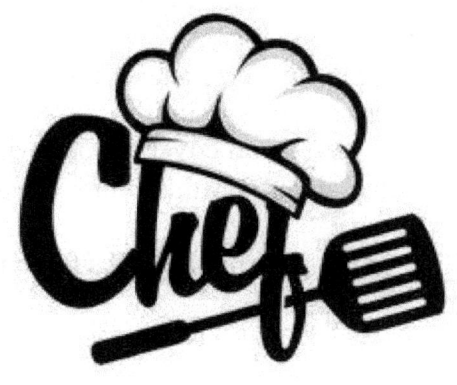

Chicken, avocado, arugula and buckwheat crackers

Preparation time: 5 minutes

Cooking time: 15 minutes

Ingredients:

- ✓ ½ avocado juice from ¼ lemon
- ✓ 1 teaspoon extra virgin olive oil
- ✓ 20 g celery, diced
- ✓ 20 g red onion, diced
- ✓ 100 g cooked chicken breast, cut into bite-sized pieces
- ✓ 2–3 buckwheat crackers (store-bought or homemade)
- ✓ 10 g rocket

Nutritional values: (1 serving)

Carbohydrates: 6 | Fat: 11 | Protein: 27 | Kcal: 200

Preparation:

- ✓ Peel the avocado then mash it with the back of a fork.

- ✓ Add lemon juice, olive oil, celery and red onion and mix well.

- ✓ Stir in the chicken. Spread the mixture over the crackers and cover with the rocket.

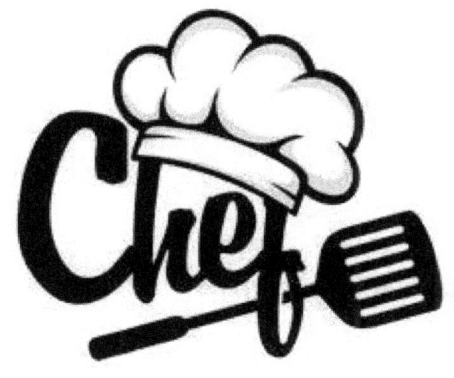

Buckwheat Gallo Pinto

(Fried eggs with seasoned buckwheat and beans)

Preparation time: 10 minutes

Cooking time: 10 minutes

Ingredients:
- ✓ 2 teaspoons of extra virgin olive oil
- ✓ 30 g diced red onion
- ✓ 30 g celery, diced
- ✓ 15 g kale (weight with stems removed), chopped
- ✓ 1 chopped chili
- ✓ 1 teaspoon paprika
- ✓ 1 teaspoon ground turmeric
- ✓ 60 g of boiled buckwheat
- ✓ 50 g canned black beans or kidney beans, drained
- ✓ 1 tbsp chopped coriander
- ✓ 2 medium-sized eggs

Nutritional values: (1 serving)

Carbohydrates: 17 | Fat: 15 | Protein: 9 | Kcal: 250

Preparation:

- ✓ Put a small saucepan over low to medium heat. Add 1 teaspoon of olive oil and saute the red onions, celery, kale, and chilies for 2-3 minutes or until tender.

- ✓ Add the spices and cook for another minute. Add the buckwheat, beans and a splash of water and fry well.

- ✓ Add the coriander. In the meantime, prepare the eggs.

- ✓ Put a pan over medium heat, add the remaining teaspoon of olive oil and fry the eggs to your liking.

- ✓ Serve over buckwheat and beans.

Chilli and turmeric Hummus

Preparation time: 10 minutes

Cooking time: -

Ingredients:

- ✓ 1 × 400 g can of chickpeas, drained
- ✓ 2 tbsp tahini
- ✓ 1 tbsp extra virgin olive oil juice
- ✓ 1 lemon
- ✓ 50 ml of water
- ✓ 1 chopped chili, chopped
- ✓ 1 teaspoon ground turmeric

Nutritional values: (2 servings)
Carbohydrates: 12 | Fat: 5 | Protein: 3 | Kcal: 80

Preparation:

- Put all ingredients in a food processor and mix for 2-3 minutes until a smooth paste is formed. Feel free to add a little more water depending on how thick you like your hummus.

Scrambled eggs with kale, red onions and tomatoes

Preparation time: 15 minutes

Cooking time: 10 minutes

Ingredients:

- ✓ 100 g extra firm tofu
- ✓ 30 g of chopped kale (weight with stems removed)
- ✓ 1 teaspoon ground turmeric
- ✓ 1 teaspoon extra virgin olive oil
- ✓ 20 g cut red onion
- ✓ 20 g cut celery
- ✓ ½ cut chili
- ✓ 5 halved cherry tomatoes
- ✓ 5 g chopped parsley

Nutritional values: (1 serving)

Carbohydrates: 5 | Fat: 9 | Protein: 13 | Kcal: 110

Preparation:

- ✓ Wrap the tofu in kitchen paper and place something heavy on top to remove any excess water.

- ✓ Steam the kale for 2-3 minutes. Mix the turmeric and some water until a light paste is formed. Put a pan over medium heat, add the olive oil then the onion, celery and chilies and sauté for 2-3 minutes.

- ✓ Crumble the tofu into bite-sized pieces and add to the pan with the cherry tomatoes then pour over the turmeric paste and mix thoroughly. Add the kale and keep stirring and frying until the tofu is browned. Add parsley and serve.

Smoked trout, curd cheese and caper crackers

Preparation time: 15 minutes

Cooking time: 10 minutes

Ingredients:

- ✓ 50 g of cottage cheese
- ✓ 1 teaspoon capers
- ✓ 1 teaspoon chopped parsley
- ✓ 20 g diced red onion
- ✓ 2–3 buckwheat crackers (store bought or homemade)
- ✓ 10 g rocket
- ✓ 75 g sliced smoked trout
- ✓ Lemon juice

Nutritional values: (1 serving)

Carbohydrates: 12 | Fat: 3 | Protein: 4 | Kcal: 80

Preparation:

- Mix the cottage cheese, capers, parsley and red onion in a bowl. Spread the mixture over the crackers and top with the rocket and smoked trout.
- Press over the lemon juice to serve.

Kale and toasted Walnut soup

Preparation time: 15 minutes

Cooking time: approx. 1 hour

Ingredients:

- ✓ 2 teaspoons of native olive oil
- ✓ 30g heard red onion
- ✓ 30 grams of heard celery
- ✓ 1 clove of heard garlic
- ✓ 1 teaspoon dried thyme
- ✓ 75 g canned or homemade white beans such as cannellini or haricot
- ✓ 500 ml vegetable broth
- ✓ 50 g kale, roughly chopped
- ✓ 4 chopped walnut halves

Nutritional values: (1 serving)

Carbohydrates: 18 | Fat: 22 | Protein: 12 | Kcal: 260

Preparation:

- ✓ In a medium saucepan, heat 1 teaspoon of olive oil over medium heat and fry the red onions, celery and garlic for 2-3 minutes. When soft, add the thyme, beans, and broth and bring to a boil.

- ✓ Simmer over low heat for 25 minutes then add the kale and cook for another 10 minutes. When all of the vegetables are cooked through, blend the mixture until smooth. You may need to add some water if your soup is too thick. If it looks very watery before mixing, just turn up the heat and let it bubble until it's thicker.

- ✓ While the soup is cooking, heat your oven to 160 ° C / Gas 3 and roast your walnuts for 10-15 minutes so they are nicely browned. Watch them carefully as they can easily switch from roasted to burnt. Serve your soup drizzled with the remaining teaspoon of olive oil and topped with the roasted walnuts.

Spicy lentils Vegetable soup

Preparation time: 10 minutes

Cooking time: 30 minutes

Ingredients:

- ✓ 1 teaspoon extra virgin olive oil plus
- ✓ 30 g red onion
- ✓ 30 g celery
- ✓ 30 g carrot
- ✓ 1 Birds Eye Chili
- ✓ 1 clove of garlic
- ✓ 1 teaspoon ground turmeric
- ✓ 1 tsp curry powder
- ✓ 500 ml vegetable broth
- ✓ 50 g red lentils
- ✓ 1 teaspoon chopped parsley

Nutritional values: (1 serving)

Carbohydrates: 14 | Fat: 7 | Protein: 8 | Kcal: 120

Preparation:

- ✓ In a small saucepan, heat the olive oil over low to medium heat and fry the onion, celery and carrot for 2-3 minutes until soft. Add the chili, garlic and spices and cook for another minute. Add vegetable stock and lentils and bring to a boil. Simmer gently for 30 minutes and stir from time to time so that nothing sticks to the bottom.

- ✓ Once the lentils have broken down and they have a nice soupy consistency, stir in the parsley and serve with a dash of extra virgin olive oil.

Sirt chicken salad

Preparation time: 15 minutes

Cooking time: -

Ingredients:

- ✓ 75 g natural yogurt juice from ¼ lemon
- ✓ 1 teaspoon chopped coriander
- ✓ 1 teaspoon ground turmeric
- ✓ ½ teaspoon mild curry powder
- ✓ 100 g cooked chicken breast, cut into bite-sized pieces
- ✓ 6 chopped walnut halves
- ✓ 1 Medjool date, finely chopped
- ✓ 20 g diced red onion
- ✓ 1 chili
- ✓ 40g arugula to serve

Nutritional values: (1 serving)

Carbohydrates: 24 | Fat: 14 | Protein: 22 | Kcal: 310

Preparation:

- Mix the yogurt, lemon juice, coriander and spices in a bowl. Add all the remaining ingredients and serve on a bed of arugula.

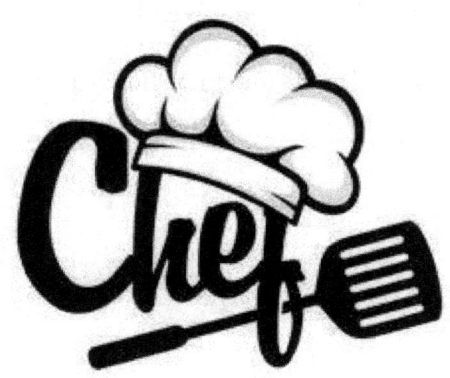

Tuna and chicory boats

Preparation time: 10 minutes

Cooking time: -

Ingredients:

- ✓ 1 × 150 g can of drained tuna (in oil or brine)
- ✓ 20 g diced red onion
- ✓ 20 g diced celery
- ✓ 1 teaspoon capers
- ✓ 1 teaspoon chopped parsley juice
- ✓ ¼ lemon
- ✓ 1 teaspoon extra virgin olive oil
- ✓ 1 head of chicory
- ✓ 5–6 chopped walnut halves

Nutritional values: (1 serving)

Carbohydrates: 18 | Fat: 25 | Protein: 26 | Kcal: 430

Preparation:

• Place the tuna in a bowl and add onion, celery, capers, parsley, lemon juice and olive oil. Mix well.

• Cut the end of the chicory head and separate the leaves. Put the tuna in as many leaves as possible and sprinkle over the chopped walnuts.

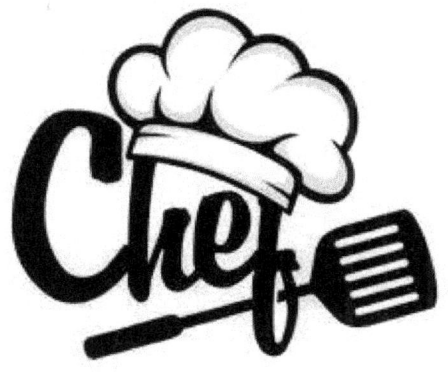

Kale, red onion and cheese frittata

Preparation time: 10 minutes

Cooking time: 25 minutes

Ingredients:

- ✓ 3 medium-sized eggs
- ✓ 1 teaspoon extra virgin olive oil
- ✓ 40 g red onion, cut
- ✓ 40 g of cut kale (weight with stems removed)
- ✓ 1 small clove of garlic
- ✓ ½ teaspoon herbs of Provence
- ✓ 1 teaspoon chopped parsley
- ✓ 20 g cheese (feta, cheddar)

Nutritional values: (1 serving)

Carbohydrates: 25 | Fat: 15 | Protein: 13 | Kcal: 260

Preparation:

- Heat the oven to 180 ° C / gas. 4. In a bowl, crack the eggs and whisk them well.
- Heat the olive oil in an ovenproof pan over low to medium heat and fry the onion, kale, and garlic for 3-4 minutes or until tender.
- Add the cooked vegetables to the egg mixture. Add herbs and parsley and stir well. You can rub or crumble the cheese into the egg as you wish.
- Turn the pan back on high heat and add the egg mixture. Let sit on the heat for 30 seconds or until the egg comes off the side of the pan. Transfer the pan to the oven. Bake for 15 minutes until the egg has set.
- If it's still a little runny in the middle, you can take it out of the oven and let it rest for 5 minutes before serving, as the residual heat will continue to cook the frittata.
- You could serve with a little arugula on top and a splash of olive oil.

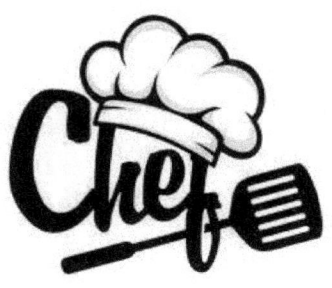

Lemon herb sardines with rocket, Avocado and caper salad

Preparation time: 15 minutes

Cooking time: -

Ingredients:

- ✓ Juice of ½ lemon
- ✓ 30 g cut red onion
- ✓ 30 g sliced celery
- ✓ ½ avocado
- ✓ 40 g rocket
- ✓ 1 teaspoon capers
- ✓ 2 chopped walnut halves
- ✓ 1 teaspoon extra virgin olive oil
- ✓ 120 g drained canned sardines (boneless, best in olive oil or brine)
- ✓ 1 tbsp chopped parsley

Nutritional values: (1 serving)

Carbohydrates: 16 | Fat: 23 | Protein: 8 | Kcal: 170

Preparation:

- Mix half of the lemon juice with the red onion and celery. Cut the avocado into slices and mix with arugula, capers, walnuts and olive oil.
- Mix the sardines with the parsley and the rest of the lemon juicethen serve them on top of the avocado and arugula mixture.

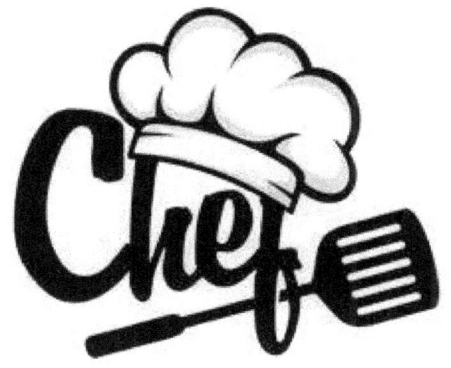

Bean seaweed salad with miso dressing

Preparation time: 10 minutes

Cooking time: -

Ingredients:

- ✓ 100 g canned or homemade mixed beans(drained)
- ✓ 5 g arame or wakame, prepared according to the instructions on the package
- ✓ 20 g cut red onion
- ✓ 30 g diced cucumber
- ✓ 20 g celery, cut
- ✓ 40 g rocket For the miso dressing
- ✓ 1 tbsp miso paste
- ✓ 1 teaspoon extra virgin olive oil
- ✓ 1 teaspoon rice vinegar
- ✓ 1 teaspoon chopped coriander
- ✓ 1 teaspoon sesame seeds

Nutritional values: (1 serving)

Carbohydrates: 13 | Fat: 11 | Protein: 3 | Kcal: 120

Preparation:

- First prepare the dressing: whisk all ingredients together and set aside. Mix all salad ingredients in a bowl except for the rocket. Mix with the miso dressing and serve on a rocket bed.

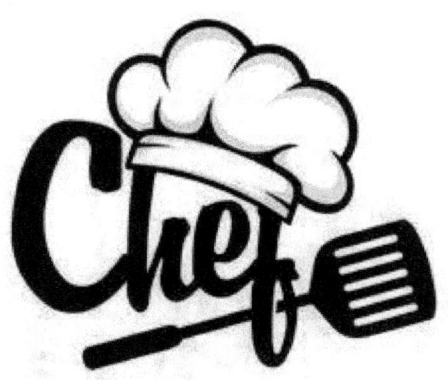

White bean salad, kale and sun-dried tomatoes

Preparation time: 15 minutes

Cooking time: -

Ingredients:

- ✓ 30 g kale (weight with stems removed), finely chopped
- ✓ 1 tbsp pumpkin seeds
- ✓ 100 g canned or homemade beans such as cannellini or haricot
- ✓ 25 g sun-dried tomatoes, finely chopped
- ✓ 1 teaspoon chopped parsley
- ✓ 20 g red onion, diced
- ✓ 20 g celery, cut
- ✓ ½ cooked beetroot, diced
- ✓ 10 g pitted black olive juice
- ✓ 1 teaspoon extra virgin olive oil
- ✓ 40 g rocket

Nutritional values: (1 serving)

Carbohydrates: 28 | Fat: 18 | Protein: 13 | Kcal: 290

Preparation:

- ✓ Steam or cook the kale for about 5 minutes until tender. Drain and set aside.

- ✓ In the meantime, roast the pumpkin seeds in a dry pan, remove them and set aside.

- ✓ Mix the beans, tomatoes, parsley, onion, celery, beetroot and olives in a bowl. Add lemon juice and olive oil and mix well.

- ✓ Stir the kale through the salad and serve on a bed of rocket sprinkled with pumpkin seeds.

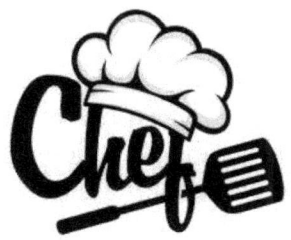

Chicken skewers with satay sauce and buckwheat

Preparation time: 15 minutes

Cooking time: 1 hour 30 minutes

Ingredients:

- ✓ 150 g chicken breast, cut into pieces
- ✓ 1 teaspoon ground turmeric
- ✓ ½ teaspoon extra virgin olive oil
- ✓ 50 g buckwheat
- ✓ 30 g kale (weight without stems removed)
- ✓ 30 g celery cut into slices
- ✓ 4 walnut halves sliced, chopped, to refine

For the sauce

- ✓ 20 g red onion
- ✓ 1 clove of garlic diced
- ✓ 1 teaspoon extra virgin olive oil chopped
- ✓ 1 tsp curry powder
- ✓ 1 teaspoon ground turmeric
- ✓ 50 ml chicken broth
- ✓ 150 ml coconut milk
- ✓ 1 tbsp walnut butter or peanut butter
- ✓ 1 tbsp chopped coriander

__Nutritional values:__ (1 serving)

Carbohydrates: 11 | Fat: 13 | Protein: 26 | Kcal: 310

Preparation:

- ✓ Mix the chicken with turmeric and olive oil and set aside to marinate - 30 minutes to 1 hour is best, but if you're short on time just leave it as long as possible.
- ✓ Cook the buckwheat according to the directions in the package and add the kale and celery for the final 5 to 7 minutes of cooking time.
- ✓ Drain. Heat the grill on a high level.
- ✓ For the sauce

- ✓ Fry the red onion and garlic in the olive oil for 2-3 minutes until tender.
- ✓ Add the spices and cook for another minute. Add the stock and coconut milk and bring to a boil, then add the walnut butter and stir.
- ✓ Reduce the heat and simmer the sauce for 8-10 minutes or until creamy and rich.
- ✓ While the sauce is cooking, thread the chicken on the skewers and place under the hot grill for 10 minutes.
- ✓ Turn it over after 5 minutes. To serve, stir the coriander through the sauce and pour over the skewers then sprinkle over the chopped walnuts.

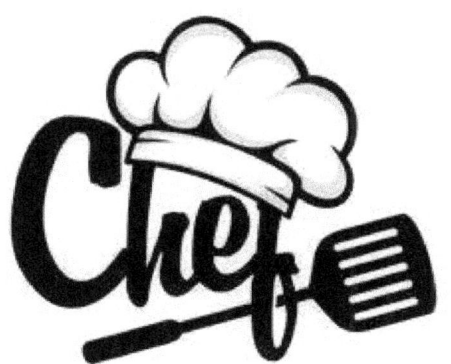

Baked Cod with Kale, Chicory and white beans

Preparation time: 10 minutes

Cooking time: 20 minutes

Ingredients:

- ✓ 150 g cod fillet
- ✓ ½ teaspoon extra virgin olive oil
- ✓ 1 teaspoon chopped parsley

For the beans

- ✓ 50 g kale, sliced, the stems removed
- ✓ 1 teaspoon extra virgin olive oil
- ✓ 30 g red onion
- ✓ 1 clove of garlic sliced
- ✓ 100 ml vegetable stock
- ✓ 75 g from the can or homemade white beans such as cannellini or haricot
- ✓ 1 head of chicory, halved lengthways and sliced

Nutritional values: (1 serving)

Carbohydrates: 16 | Fat: 26 | Protein: 31 | Kcal: 430

Preparation:

- ✓ Heat the oven to 200 ° C / gas. 6. Line a small baking sheet with parchment paper.
- ✓ Steam or cook the kale for 5–7 minutes until tender, then set aside. Rub the fish with olive oil and parsley, place on the prepared tray and bake in the oven for 10 minutes.
- ✓ In the meantime, heat the olive oil in a small saucepan over low to medium heat and fry the red onion and garlic for 2-3 minutes until tender.
- ✓ Add the stock and beans and bring to a boil. Add the chicory and cook on low to medium heat for a few more minutes.
- ✓ Be careful not to cook it too long. Stir the kale through the mixture and serve with the fish.

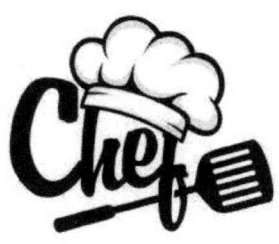

Chicory made from tofu and chili with arugula walnut salad

Preparation time: 10 minutes

Cooking time: 30 minutes

Ingredients:

- ✓ 1 teaspoon extra virgin olive oil
- ✓ 30 g red onion, diced
- ✓ 30 g celery, diced
- ✓ 1 clove of garlic, chopped
- ✓ 1 chili, chopped
- ✓ 1 teaspoon thyme (fresh or dried)
- ✓ 1 × 400 g can of tomatoes
- ✓ 150 g silken tofu, cut into small cubes
- ✓ 1 tbsp chopped parsley
- ✓ 2 heads of chicory, quartered lengthways

For the salad

- ✓ 35 g rocket
- ✓ 1 teaspoon capers
- ✓ 6 walnut halves, chopped
- ✓ 1 teaspoon extra virgin olive oil
- ✓ 1 tsp balsamic vinegar

Nutritional values : (1 serving)

Carbohydrates: 11 | Fat: 21 | Protein: 26 | Kcal: 330

Preparation:

- Preheat the oven to 200 ° C / gas. 6. In a medium saucepan, heat the olive

oil over medium heat and cook the red onions, celery, garlic, chilies and thyme for 2-3 minutes or until tender.
- Add tomatoes and bring to a boil. Wash the can with a little water and pour the liquid into the pan.
- Let simmer for 10–15 minutes. Add the tofu and parsley, being careful not to break the tofu.
- Place the chicory in a baking dish. Turn the oven to 220 ° C / gas. 7th
- Pour the hot sauce over the chicory and bake for 8-10 minutes, until the chicory is wilted and cooked.
- In the meantime, mix all the ingredients for the salad in a bowl and serve with the chicory.

Asian marinated tofu with Satay sauce and buckwheat with Arame

Preparation time: 15 minutes

Cooking time: 35 minutes

Ingredients:

- ✓ 150 g firm tofu
- ✓ ½ teaspoon extra virgin olive oil
- ✓ 1 teaspoon tamari (or soy sauce)
- ✓ 1 teaspoon ground turmeric
- ✓ 50 g buckwheat
- ✓ 5 g arame
- ✓ 2 chopped walnut halves for garnish (optional)

For the sauce
- ✓ 20 g red onion,
- ✓ 1 garlic diced clove, chopped
- ✓ 1 teaspoon extra virgin olive oil
- ✓ 1 teaspoon ground turmeric
- ✓ 1 tsp curry powder
- ✓ 50 ml vegetable broth
- ✓ 150 ml coconut milk
- ✓ 1 tbsp walnut butter or peanut butter
- ✓ 1 tbsp chopped coriander

Nutritional values: (1 serving)
Carbohydrates: 23 | Fat: 35 | Protein: 31 | Kcal: 560

Preparation:

- ✓ Drain the tofu and pat dry with kitchen paper. Cut the tofu into bite-sized pieces and mix with olive oil, tamari and turmeric.
- ✓ Set aside for marinating. Boil the buckwheat and prepare the arame according to the instructions on their packet.
- ✓ Then drain them and mix them together. Heat the grill on a high level. For the sauce, fry the red onion and garlic in the olive oil for 2-3 minutes until they are soft.
- ✓ Add the spices and cook for another minute. Add the stock and coconut milk and bring to a boil, then add the walnut butter and stir.
- ✓ Reduce the heat and cook the sauce for 8-10 minutes or until creamy and rich. Then stir in the coriander.
- ✓ Thread the tofu pieces on a skewer and grill for 8 to 10 minutes.
- ✓ Then turn it halfway once. They're done when they're nicely tanned. • Serve the tofu on a bed of buckwheat and drizzle the sauce over it.

✓ Sprinkle over the chopped walnuts if used.

Tuna noodles

Preparation time: 10 minutes

Cooking time: 15 minutes

Ingredients:

- ✓ 75 g buckwheat noodles
- ✓ 30 g red onion
- ✓ 30 g celery cut into slices
- ✓ 30 g sliced kale (weight without stems), finely chopped
- ✓ 1 clove of garlic, chopped
- ✓ 1 teaspoon herbs of Provence
- ✓ 1 teaspoon extra virgin olive oil 100 ml vegetable broth
- ✓ 1 tbsp chopped parsley
- ✓ 1 teaspoon capers
- ✓ 1 × 150 g can of tuna (in oil or salt solution), drained

Nutritional values: (1 serving)

Carbohydrates: 8 | Fat: 12 | Protein: 21 | Kcal: 260

Preparation:

- ✓ Cook the pasta according to the instructions in the package. In the meantime, cook the onion, celery, kale, garlic, and dried herbs in olive oil over low to medium heat for 3 to 4 minutes until tender.
- ✓ Add the broth and cook for a few more minutes on a similar heat. When all the vegetables are cooked to your satisfaction, stir in the parsley, capers and tuna. Add the cooked noodles, heat everything through and serve.

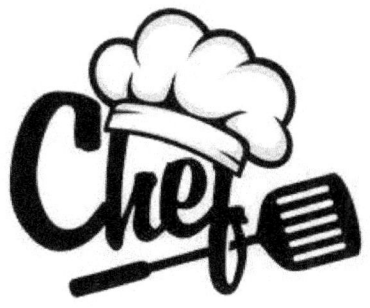

Fried Thai Prawns

Preparation time: 10 minutes
Cooking time: 10 minutes

Ingredients:
- ✓ 50 g buckwheat
- ✓ 1 teaspoon ground turmeric
- ✓ 125 g chicken breast, sliced or cut into bite-sized pieces or raw king prawns, peeled and deveined
- ✓ 40 g celery, cut diagonally into 1 cm slices
- ✓ 25 g of kale (weight with stems removed), cut
- ✓ 100 ml chicken broth or vegetable broth
- ✓ 4–5 basil leaves

For the stir-fry dishes
- ✓ 30 g red onion
- ✓ 1 lemongrass stalk chopped
- ✓ 1 clove of garlic chopped
- ✓ 1 chili, chopped
- ✓ 1 teaspoon ground turmeric
- ✓ 1 teaspoon ground cumin
- ✓ 1 cm fresh ginger chopped, chopped
- ✓ 1 teaspoon extra virgin olive oil
- ✓ 1 tbsp chopped parsley
- ✓ 1 teaspoon fish sauce, soy sauce or tamari

Nutritional values: (1 serving)
Carbohydrates: 8 | Fat: 10 | Protein: 25 | Kcal: 230

Preparation:

• Cook the buckwheat according to the instructions on the package, stirring the turmeric into the water.
• In the meantime, put all the ingredients in the paste in a food processor and flash until you get a smooth paste.
• If you don't have a food processor, just chop everything as finely as you can and mix well.
• Heat the paste in a pan over medium heat. Add the chicken or shrimp along with the celery and kale and cook for 4 to 5 minutes, or until the chicken or shrimp is cooked through.
• Add the broth and cook for another 1-2 minutes. Halve the basil leaves and add to the pan. Serve with the buckwheat.

Grilled turkey schnitzel with Walnut, herb and cheddar crust

Preparation time: 10 minutes

Cooking time: 10 minutes

Ingredients:
- ✓ 150 g turkey schnitzel or turkey breast steak
- ✓ ½ teaspoon extra virgin olive oil
- ✓ 10 g cheddar cheese, grated
- ✓ 1 tbsp chopped parsley
- ✓ 10 g red onion, diced
- ✓ 10 g walnuts, chopped
- ✓ Juice of ¼ lemon

For the salad
- ✓ 100 g tomato slices
- ✓ 40 g rocket
- ✓ 20 g red onions, cut
- ✓ 1 teaspoon capers
- ✓ 30 g celery, cut
- ✓ 1 teaspoon extra virgin olive oil
- ✓ 1 tsp balsamic vinegar

Nutritional values: (1 serving)

Carbohydrates: 9 | Fat: 17 | Protein: 27 | Kcal: 330

Preparation:

- ✓ Heat the grill on a high level. Rub the turkey with the olive oil, place on a baking sheet and grill for 4 minutes on each side.

- ✓ In a small bowl, mix the cheese with parsley, red onions and walnuts. Put all the ingredients for the salad together in a separate bowl.

- ✓ When the turkey is cooked through, cover one side with the cheese mixture and place it back on the grill for 2-3 minutes, or until the cheese and walnuts begin to brown.

- ✓ Squeeze the lemon juice over the schnitzel and serve with the salad.

Lamb Date Kofta with Tzatziki, rocket and Chili buckwheat

Preparation time: 15 minutes

Cooking time: 45 minutes

Ingredients:
- ✓ 1 Medjool dates, chopped
- ✓ 1 teaspoon ground turmeric
- ✓ 1 teaspoon ground cumin
- ✓ 20 g red onion
- ✓ 1 teaspoon chopped parsley
- ✓ 1 medium egg yolk
- ✓ 1 small clove of garlic
- ✓ 150 g minced lamb

For the buckwheat
- ✓ 30 g buckwheat
- ✓ 1 chili, chopped
- ✓ 1 teaspoon chopped parsley

For the tzatziki
- ✓ 50 g natural yogurt
- ✓ 20 g cucumber, grated
- ✓ ½ teaspoon dried or fresh mint juice (optional)
- ✓ ¼ lemon

For the salad
- ✓ 50 g tomato, diced
- ✓ 30 g rocket
- ✓ 1 teaspoon extra virgin olive oil juice
- ✓ ¼ lemon

Nutritional values: (1 serving)

Carbohydrates: 19 | Fat: 23 | Protein: 25 | Kcal: 420

Preparation:

• To make the kofta, put all of the ingredients except the ground beef in a food processor and blend until you have a smooth paste. Remove this paste and knead it into the lamb. Shape the meat into two sausages and refrigerate for 30 minutes before cooking. Cook the buckwheat according to the instructions on the package.

• For the tzatziki, simply mix all the ingredients together and set aside.

Heat the grill on a high level.

• Place your Kofta under the grill for 8-10 minutes, turning it from time to time until it is nicely browned and cooked through.

• In the meantime, add the chopped chillies and parsley to the buckwheat and stir.

- For the salad, simply mix all the ingredients in a bowl. Serve all finished items together.

Beef burger with Sweet potato fries

Preparation time: 15 minutes

Cooking time: 35 minutes

Ingredients:
- ✓ 125 g lean ground beef (5 percent fat)
- ✓ 15 g red onion, finely chopped
- ✓ 1 teaspoon finely chopped parsley
- ✓ 1 teaspoon extra virgin olive oil

For the fries
- ✓ 150 g sweet potatoes
- ✓ 1 teaspoon extra virgin olive oil
- ✓ 1 teaspoon dried rosemary
- ✓ 1 clove of garlic, unpeeled

For serving
- ✓ 10 g cheddar cheese, sliced or grated
- ✓ 150 g red onion, cut into rings
- ✓ 30 g tomato, cut 10 g rocket 1 pickle (optional)

Nutritional values: (1 serving)
Carbohydrates: 21 | Fat: 31 | Protein: 28 | Kcal: 510

Preparation:
- Heat the oven to 220 ° C / gas. 7. Make the fries first.
- Peel the sweet potato and cut into 1 cm thick French fries. Mix them with olive oil, rosemary and clove of garlic.
- Place on a baking sheet and cook for 30 minutes until crispy.
- For the burger, mix the onion and parsley with the ground beef. If you have cookie cutters, you can shape your burger using the largest cookie cutter in the set.
- Otherwise, just use your hands to make a nice, even pie. Heat a pan over medium heat, add the olive oil and place the burger on one side of the pan and the onion rings on the other.
- Cook the burger for 6 minutes on each side, making sure it is done. Fry the onion rings to taste.
- When the burger is cooked, pour the cheese and red onion on top and place in the hot oven for a minute to melt the cheese.
- Take out the tomatoes, rocket and pickles and place on top. Serve with the fries.

Salmon tartare with rocket salad

Preparation time: 15 minutes

Cooking time: 35 minutes

Ingredients:
- ✓ 125 g skinless salmon fillet without bones
- ✓ 20 g red onion
- ✓ 1 teaspoon capers
- ✓ 1 teaspoon extra virgin olive oil
- ✓ 1 tbsp chopped parsley juice made from ¼ lemon salt and pepper

For the salad
- ✓ 40 g rocket 6
- ✓ Walnut halves, chopped
- ✓ 40 g celery, cut
- ✓ 1 teaspoon extra virgin olive oil
- ✓ 1 tsp balsamic vinegar

Nutritional values: (1 serving)

Carbohydrates: 15 | Fat: 25 | Protein: 23 | Kcal: 390

Preparation:

- Halve the salmon fillet. Next, cut each half into thin strips and chop them into small cubes.
- Chop the red onions and capers as small as possible and mix them with the salmon.
- If you have a small food processor, you can use this to chop it up.
- Mix with olive oil, parsley and a little salt and pepper. Mix all the ingredients for the salad and serve with the salmon on top.
- Squeeze the lemon juice over the salmon and you're good to go (don't add the lemon juice before serving as it will react with the raw fish and start cooking).

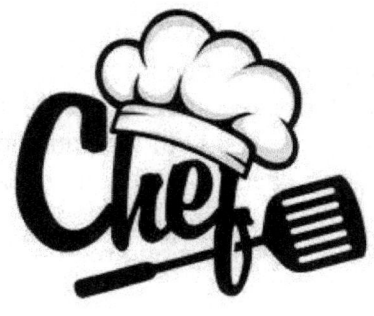

Stuffed portobello mushroom with braised celery

Preparation time: 15 minutes

Cooking time: 1 hour 20 minutes

Ingredients:
- ✓ 50 g canned or homemade white beans such as cannellini or haricot
- ✓ 1 teaspoon parsley
- ✓ 2 walnut halves
- ✓ 1 tbsp sunflower seeds
- ✓ 1 teaspoon extra virgin olive oil
- ✓ 30 g red onion, cut
- ✓ 20 g of kale (weight with stems removed), cut
- ✓ 1 clove of garlic, chopped
- ✓ 1 large portobello mushroom 20 g rocket for serving

For the celery
- ✓ 3-4 celery stalks
- ✓ Halve 350 ml vegetable stock
- ✓ 1 teaspoon dried thyme or
- ✓ 1 sprig of fresh thyme
- ✓ 1 clove of garlic
- ✓ teaspoon ground turmeric

Nutritional values: (1 serving)

Carbohydrates: 23 | Fat: 15 | Protein: 7 | Kcal: 250

Preparation:

- Preheat the oven to 180 ° C / gas 4. For the celery, simply place all the ingredients in an ovenproof bowl. Cover with a lid or foil and bake for 30 to 40 minutes until tender.
- While the celery is cooking, prepare your mushroom so that it goes in the oven for the last 20 minutes of the celery cook time.
- For filling
- Mix the beans, parsley and walnuts together in a food processor.
- If you don't have a food processor, simply mash the beans with the back of a fork and chop the parsley and walnuts as small as possible.
- Fold in the sunflower seeds. Heat the olive oil in a small pan and gently cook the red onion, kale and garlic until soft.
- Remove from heat and stir in the bean mixture. Fill the mushroom with it and place on a baking sheet.
- Put in the oven and bake with the celery for the last 20-25 minutes. The top of the mushroom should be nicely browned.
- Serve the mushrooms with braised celery and arugula.

Arame and miso meatballs with crispy ginger kale

Preparation time: 15 minutes

Cooking time: 45 minutes

Ingredients:
- ✓ 5 g arame
- ✓ 1 clove of garlic, chopped
- ✓ 20 g red onion, cut
- ✓ 2 teaspoons of extra virgin olive oil
- ✓ 75 g canned or homemade white beans such as cannellini or haricot
- ✓ 150 g silken tofu
- ✓ 20 g miso paste
- ✓ 1 tbsp chopped coriander
- ✓ 2 tbsp sesame seeds

For the kale
- ✓ 1 teaspoon extra virgin olive oil
- ✓ 1 cm fresh ginger, chopped
- ✓ 80 g kale (weight with stems removed), chopped

Nutritional values: (1 serving)

Carbohydrates: 21 | Fat: 6 | Protein: 9 | Kcal: 150

Preparation:

- Heat the oven to 180 ° C / gas. 4. Make the kale first: rub in the olive oil and ginger, place on a tray, and bake for 25-30 minutes.
- Turn it every 10 minutes to make sure it cooks evenly. For the meatballs, prepare the arame according to the package instructions.
- Gently fry the garlic and red onion in 1 teaspoon of olive oil for 2-3 minutes.
- Pat the beans and tofu dry with kitchen paper and place in a food processor with miso and coriander. Mix to a paste.
- Drain the arame and dry it completely before stirring it into the bean mixture.
- Shape into small patties and roll up the sesame seeds. Fry the meatballs in the remaining teaspoon of olive oil over medium heat for 2-3 minutes on each side.
- They should get a nice golden brown. Serve with the kale.

Phase 2

Welcome to phase 2 of the sirtfood diet. As good as the results of phase 1 are, what really counts is the long-term implementation of a sirtfood-rich diet. That means making it everyday. Remember that sirtfoods are so much more than just weight loss.

By looking for a sustainable and long-term way to eat, sirtfoods are a culinary ticket to lifelong health and wellbeing. And honestly, who's going to turn down the opportunity to feel great just by eating deliciously?

What is the magic formula for success?

It's actually very simple. Just eat what you want, but with a big sirt food touch. It's not about counting the calories, the fats, or the carbohydrates. Long-term success can only be achieved if we focus on what we're getting from eating on our plates, not what you should lose weight.

A way of eating that you know is good for you every delicious sip. On the whole, I recommend that you base your daily diet on:

- ✓ *3 × sirtfood-rich meals*
- ✓ *1 × sirtfood green juice or smoothie*
- ✓ *1 × sirtfood snack (optional)*

A daily green sirtfood juice that is best taken when getting up before breakfast. Then it's all about balanced breakfast, lunch and dinner and, if necessary, a snack inspired by sirtfood.

BREAKFAST

Sirt cereal

Preparation time: 15 minutes

Cooking time: 1 hour 20 minutes

Ingredients:

- ✓ 50 g coconut oil
- ✓ 150 ml clear honey
- ✓ 1 tbsp ground turmeric
- ✓ 100 g oats (use certified gluten-free oats if you're avoiding gluten)
- ✓ 250 g buckwheat flakes
- ✓ 100 g walnuts, chopped
- ✓ 50 g pecans, chopped
- ✓ 50 g flaked almonds
- ✓ 30 g pumpkin seeds
- ✓ 30 g sunflower seeds and 50 g cocoa nibs

Nutritional values: (2 -3 servings)

Carbohydrates: 28 | Fat: 7 | Protein: 6 | Kcal: 220

Preparation:

- ✓ Heat your oven to 160 ° C / gas 3. In a small saucepan, melt the coconut oil and honey over low heat and then stir in the turmeric. Mix well to make sure no lumps are formed. Mix all dry ingredients in a bowl and stir in the oil and honey.

- ✓ Make sure they combine well then transfer them to a non-stick baking sheet or one lined with parchment paper.

- ✓ Bake for 35–40 minutes, stirring for half the cooking time. Once it's a nice golden color, remove it and let it cool on the baking sheet before storing in an airtight container for up to two months.

Sirt breakfast bar

Preparation time: 15 minutes
Cooking time: approx. 2 hours

Ingredients:

- ✓ 150 g pitted Medjool dates, chopped
- ✓ 150 g walnut butter
- ✓ 50 g thick honey
- ✓ 375 g sirtfood muesli

Nutritional values: *(10 servings)*
Carbohydrates: 23 | Fat: 5 | Protein: 3 | Kcal: 140

Preparation:

- ✓ Put the dates, walnut butter, and honey in a food processor and blend until you have a nice paste. This can take some time as the dates won't be crushed and you will have to scrape the sides of the bowl a few times. Transfer the paste to a mixing bowl and stir the granola, making sure it is well mixed. If you squeeze a lump of the mixture in your hand, it should stay firm.

- ✓ Line a 25 × 18 cm baking pan with parchment paper and spoon the mixture into it. Use your hands or the back of a spoon to spread it around the can as evenly as possible then blot firmly to make sure the bars stay in one piece as you cut. Alternatively, you can shape the mixture into bite-sized balls.

- ✓ Chill at least 2 hours before attempting to cut the mixture into about 10 bars. You can then store them in an airtight container in the refrigerator for up to two weeks.

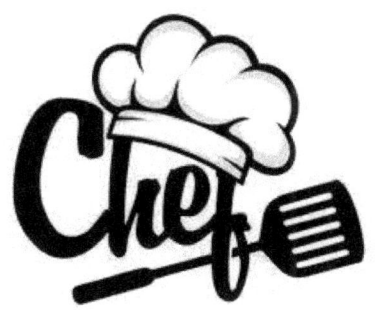

Sirt cocoa pops

Preparation time: 10 minutes

Cooking time: 25 minutes

Ingredients:
- ✓ 100 g corn
- ✓ 1 extra virgin olive oil or melted coconut oil

For covering
- ✓ 50 g walnuts, chopped
- ✓ 50 g sunflower seeds
- ✓ 50 g buckwheat flakes
- ✓ 35 g cocoa nibs

For serving
- ✓ 1 teaspoon cocoa powder (100 percent)
- ✓ 1 Medjool date, finely chopped
- ✓ 200 ml milk or dairy-free alternative

Nutritional values: (10 servings)

Carbohydrates: 21 | Fat: 14 | Protein: 3 | Kcal: 230

Preparation:

- Heat the oven to 160 ° C / gas 3. Place a heavy pan with a tightly fitting lid over medium heat.
- Mix the corn and oil, pour the mixture into the hot pan and cover with the lid. Shake the pan to get the corn moving in it.
- Once it starts to pop, turn up the heat and shake the pan for as long as you can while the lid is still on.
- Once the popping has settled down to about 2 to 3 seconds between pops, remove the pan from the heat and empty it into a bowl.
- Discard any kernels that have not popped, allow to cool completely, then transfer to an airtight container and store for up to a week.
- For the topping, place the walnuts and sunflower seeds in a small baking sheet and roast in the oven for 15 minutes. Transfer to a bowl and mix with the buckwheat and cocoa nibs.
- Let it cool completely and then store it in an airtight container for up to 1 month. The corn and topping should be stored separately to ensure even distribution when serving.
- To serve, add 1–2 tablespoons of toppings and 10 g of popcorn to a bowl. Stir the cocoa powder and date into the milk then pour it over the grain.

Sirt fruit bowl

Preparation time: 15 minutes

Cooking time: -

Ingredients:
- ✓ 40 g (10) raspberries
- ✓ 60 g (10) red / black grapes, halved
- ✓ 80 g (1 medium) plum, chopped
- ✓ 60 g (½ medium)
- ✓ Apple, cut
- ✓ 50 g (2 medium) peeled strawberries, chopped
- ✓ Juice of ¼ lemon
- ✓ 100 g Greek yogurt
- ✓ 5 walnut halves, mashed

Nutritional values: (1 serving)

Carbohydrates: 24 | Fat: 17 | Protein: 3 | Kcal: 180

Preparation:

- ✓ Put all the fruits in a bowl. Squeeze the lemon juice over it and mix well. Pour over the Greek yogurt, sprinkle the chopped walnuts on top and serve.

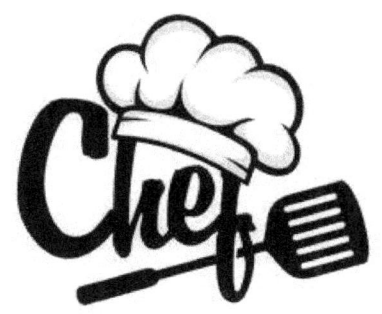

Grilled sausages with fried Onions and scrambled eggs with herbs

Preparation time: 10 minutes

Cooking time: 20 minutes

Ingredients:
- ✓ 2 lean pork or beef sausages
- ✓ 2 eggs
- ✓ 1 teaspoon chopped parsley
- ✓ 1 teaspoon chopped chives
- ✓ 25 ml milk or dairy-free alternative
- ✓ 1 teaspoon extra virgin olive oil
- ✓ 60 g red onion
- ✓ 1 teaspoon dried thyme

<u>Nutritional values:</u> (1 serving)

Carbohydrates: 24 | Fat: 27 | Protein: 15 | Kcal: 420

Preparation:

- ✓ Heat a grill on the highest setting. Grill the sausages for 8 to 10 minutes, turning them from time to time until they are brownednicely all over.

- ✓ Whisk eggs, parsley, chives and milk together. Put ½ teaspoon of olive oil in a small saucepan over medium heat, add the egg mixture and cook gently until you have a nice scrambled egg.

- ✓ In the meantime, put the remaining ½ teaspoon of olive oil in a small pan over medium heat and fry the onion and thyme for 3-4 minutes until brown.

- ✓ Stack the eggs on a plate and cover with the sausages and onions.

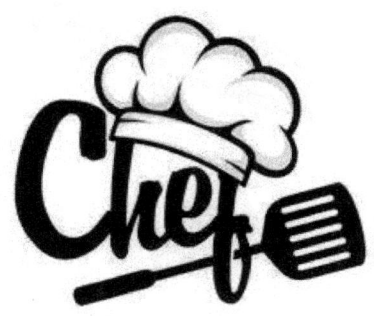

Smoked salmon, arugula and Capers on buckwheat crackers

Preparation time: 10 minutes
Cooking time: -

Ingredients:
- ✓ 1 teaspoon capers
- ✓ 60 g Greek yogurt
- ✓ 1 tbsp chopped parsley
- ✓ 10 g red onion, thinly sliced
- ✓ Buckwheat crackers
- ✓ 75 g smoked salmon
- ✓ 20 g rocket juice from ¼ lemon

Nutritional values: (1 serving)

Carbohydrates: 15 | Fat: 7 | Protein: 3 | Kcal: 120

Preparation:

- ✓ • Mix capers, yoghurt, parsley and onion in a bowl. Spread the mixture over your crackers and top with the smoked salmon and arugula. Finally, squeeze out some lemon juice.

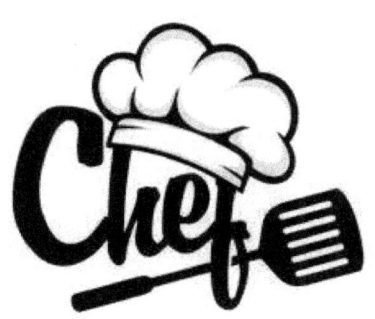

Baked Kipper with Kale and poached eggs

Preparation time: 10 minutes

Cooking time: 20 minutes

Ingredients:

- ✓ 1 tipper 1 tsp
- ✓ extra virgin olive oil
- ✓ 1 teaspoon chopped parsley
- ✓ 50 g kale, chopped
- ✓ A few drops of vinegar
- ✓ 1 medium egg
- ✓ 1 lemon wedge

Nutritional values: (1 serving)

Carbohydrates: 11 | Fat: 17 | Protein: 33 | Kcal: 340

Preparation:

- Preheat your oven to 200 ° C / gas 6. In the meantime, bring 2 small pots of water to a boil.
- If necessary, cut the head and tail off your kipper and place the skin-side down on a piece of foil.
- Pour the olive oil and parsley over the kipper and wrap the foil around it. Place the kale in a pan of boiling water and simmer for 5 minutes or until tender.
- Drain and keep warm. Put a few drops of vinegar in the other pan with boiling water and let the heat simmer.
- Stir the water clockwise and then crack your egg in half. An egg with a solid white and liquid yolk takes 2 to 3 minutes, depending on its freshness.
- Remove with a slotted spoon and drain on kitchen paper.
- Serve the egg on top of the kipper with the kale aside, or however you'd like.

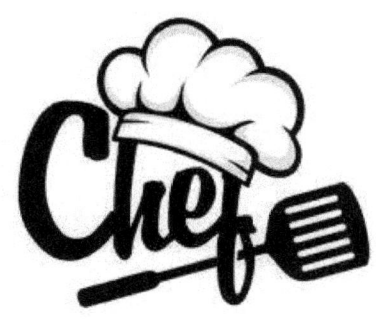

Poached egg with rocket, Asparagus and bacon

Preparation time: 5 minutes

Cooking time: 15 minutes

Ingredients:
- ✓ 2 slices of striped or bacon back
- ✓ 6 asparagus spears,
- ✓ a few drops of vinegar
- ✓ 2 eggs
- ✓ 10 g rocket
- ✓ 1 teaspoon extra virgin olive oil

Nutritional values: (1 serving)

Carbohydrates: 11 | Fat: 17 | Protein: 33 | Kcal: 340

Preparation:

- ✓ Heat a grill on the highest setting. In the meantime, bring 2 small pots of water to the boil.
- ✓ Once the grill is hot, grill your bacon until the fat is crispy - it should take 4 to 5 minutes.
- ✓ Put the asparagus spears in a pan of boiling water and cook for 2-3 minutes until tender.
- ✓ Put a few drops of vinegar in the other pan with boiling water and let the heat simmer.
- ✓ Stir the water clockwise and then crack an egg in the middle. An egg with a solid white and liquid yolk takes 2 to 3 minutes, depending on its freshness.
- ✓ Remove with a slotted spoon and drain on kitchen paper. Cook the second egg in the same way.
- ✓ Place the eggs on the asparagus, cover with the crispy bacon and rocket and drizzle over the olive oil.

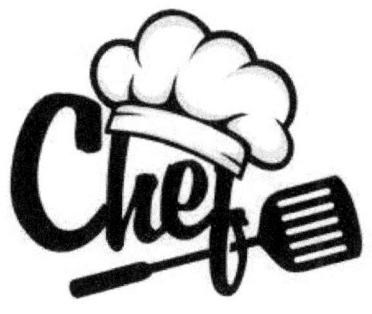

Black currants and oat yogurt

Preparation time: 10 minutes
Cooking time: -
241 calories

Ingredients:
- ✓ 100 g black currants, washed and stems removed
- ✓ 2 tbsp powdered sugar + 100 ml water
- ✓ 200 g natural yogurt
- ✓ 40 g jumbo oats

Portioning: (2 portions)

Preparation:
1. Put the black currants, sugar and water in a small pan and bring to a boil. Reduce the heat slightly, simmer vigorously, and continue cooking for 5 minutes.
2. Turn off the stove and let it cool down. The blackcurrant compote can now be refrigerated until it is used. Place the yogurt and oats in a large bowl and stir together. Divide the blackcurrant compote between two bowls and top with yogurt and oats. Use a cocktail stick to toss the compote through the yogurt.

Green omelette

Preparation time: 10 minutes
Cooking time: -
234 calories

Ingredients:
- ✓ 1 shallot, peeled and finely chopped
- ✓ 2 large eggs, at room temperature
- ✓ Handful (20 g) arugula leaves
- ✓ Small handful (10 g) parsley, finely chopped
- ✓ Salt and freshly ground black pepper

Portioning: (2 portions)

Preparation:
1. • In a wide pan, heat the oil over medium heat and gently fry the shallot for 5 minutes. Turn up the heat a little and cook for another 2 minutes. 2 In a bowl or cup, whisk the eggs well with a fork. Spread the shallot evenly in the pan before adding the eggs. Tilt the pan slightly on each side so that the egg is evenly distributed.
2. • Cook for about a minute before the sides of the omelette are raised and molten egg slides into the bottom of the pan. Immediately sprinkle over the rocket and parsley and season generously with salt and pepper.
3. • 3 After cooking, the top of the omelette is still soft, but not runny, and the base is just beginning to brown. Put on a plate and enjoy immediately.

Choc Chip Muesli

Preparation time: 30 minutes
Cooking time: -
244 calories

Ingredients:
- ✓ 200 g jumbo oats
- ✓ 50 g pecans, roughly chopped
- ✓ 3 tbsp light olive oil
- ✓ 20 g butter
- ✓ 1 tbsp dark brown sugar
- ✓ 2 tbsp rice malt syrup
- ✓ 60 g high quality (70%) dark chocolate chips

Portioning: (8 servings)

Preparation:
1. Preheat the oven to 160 ° C (140 ° C fan / gas 3). Line a large baking sheet with a silicone sheet or parchment paper.

2. Mix oats and pecans in a large bowl. In a small non-stick pan, carefully heat the olive oil, butter, brown sugar, and rice malt syrup until the butter has melted and the sugar and syrup have dissolved. Do not let cook.

3. Pour the syrup over the oats and stir thoroughly until the oats are completely covered. 3 Spread the granola on the baking sheet and spread it into the corners.

4. Leave lumps of mixture spaced apart instead of evenly distributed. Bake in the oven for 20 minutes, until the edges are golden brown. Take out of the oven and let cool completely on the tray.

5. After cooling, break up larger lumps on the tray with your fingers and mix in the chocolate chips. Scoop or pour the granola into an airtight glass. The muesli can be kept for at least 2 weeks.

Raspberry currant jelly

Preparation time: 15 minutes
Cooking time: -
76 calories

Ingredients:
- ✓ 100 g raspberries, washed
- ✓ 2 sheets of gelatin
- ✓ 100 g black currants, washed and stems removed
- ✓ 2 tbsp granulated sugar
- ✓ 300 ml of water

Portioning: (2 portions)

Preparation:
1. Arrange the raspberries in two serving dishes / glasses / tins. Place the gelatin sheets in a bowl of cold water to soften them.

2. Put the black currants with sugar and 100 ml water in a small pan and bring to the boil. Simmer vigorously for 5 minutes and then remove from heat. Let stand for 2 minutes.

3. Squeeze any excess water out of the gelatin sheets and add them to the saucepan. Stir until everything is completely dissolved then stir in the rest of the water. Pour the liquid into the prepared dishes and cool. The jellies should be ready in about 3-4 hours or overnight.

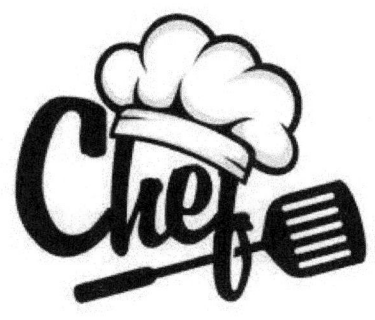

Apple pancakes with Currant compote

Preparation time: 10 minutes
Cooking time: 10 minutes
337 calories

Ingredients:

- ✓ 75 g porridge
- ✓ 125 g flour
- ✓ 1 teaspoon Baking powder
- ✓ 2 tbsp powdered sugar
- ✓ pinch of salt
- ✓ 2 apples, peeled, pitted and cut into small pieces
- ✓ 300 ml of skimmed milk
- ✓ 2 egg whites
- ✓ 2 teaspoons of light olive oil

For the compote:

- ✓ 120 g black currants, washed and stems removed
- ✓ 2 tbsp powdered sugar
- ✓ 3 tablespoons water

Portioning: (4 servings)

Preparation:

1. Make the compote first. Put the black currants, sugar and water in a small pan. Bring to a boil and cook for 10–15 minutes.
2. Put the oats, flour, baking powder, powdered sugar, and salt in a large bowl and mix well. Stir in the apple and whisk the milk one at a time until a smooth mixture is formed. Whisk the egg white until stiff and fold into the pancake batter. Transfer the batter to a jug.
3. Heat ½ teaspoon oil in a non-stick pan over medium to high heat and pour in about a quarter of the batter. Cook until golden brown on both sides. Remove and repeat to make four pancakes.
4. Serve the pancakes with the drizzled black currant compote.

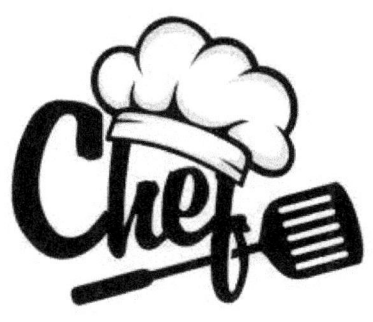

MEALS

Sirt smoked mackerel pie with celery sticks

Preparation time: 15 minutes

Cooking time: -

Ingredients:
- ✓ 1 smoked mackerel fillet (80–90 g), peeled
- ✓ 1 tbsp chopped parsley
- ✓ 1 teaspoon extra virgin olive oil
- ✓ 1 tbsp crème fraiche
- ✓ 1 tbsp cream cheese
- ✓ Pinch of freshly ground black cayenne pepper
- ✓ ¼ - ½ lemon juice, depending on taste
- ✓ 2–3 stalks of celery, depending on size

Nutritional values: (1 serving)
Carbohydrates: 16 | Fat: 13 | Protein: 7 | Kcal: 230

Preparation:

• Place three quarters of the fish in a food processor. Add the remaining ingredients except for the celery and blend until you have a smooth paste.

• Place in a bowl and peel the rest of the fish in the pie to get some texture. Cut the celery into 5 cm pieces and serve with the pie.

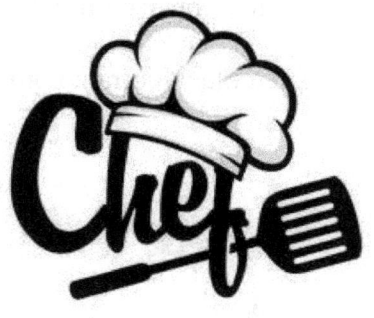

Tuna Niçoise salad

Preparation time: 10 minutes

Cooking time: 20 minutes

Ingredients:
- ✓ 50 g green beans
- ✓ 1 medium egg
- ✓ 20 g celery, diced
- ✓ 50 g cherry tomatoes, halved
- ✓ 20 g red onion, thinly sliced
- ✓ 15 g small black olives
- ✓ 1 teaspoon chopped parsley
- ✓ 2 teaspoons of extra virgin olive oil
- ✓ ½ tsp white wine vinegar
- ✓ 20 g rocket
- ✓ 1 × 150 g can of tuna (in oil or brine), depending on your taste Juice of ¼ - ½ lemon

Nutritional values: (1 serving)

Carbohydrates: 6 | Fat: 6 | Protein: 19 | Kcal: 170

Preparation:

- Bring a small saucepan of water to a boil. Once cooked, cook the beans for 3-6 minutes, depending on how crispy they are.
- Then remove with a slotted spoon and set aside. Boil the egg in the same water. If you come straight out of the fridge and let the egg simmer for 7 minutes, you will get a firm white and slightly runny yolk.
- Cook a full 10 minutes if you prefer a firm yolk. Once the time is up, place the egg under cold running water until cool enough, then peel it and set it aside.
- Mix the celery, tomatoes, onions, olives, beans and parsley with the olive oil and vinegar.
- Put this salad on top of the arugula. Cut the egg into quarters and add them, then peel the tuna meat around the plate.
- Finally squeeze some lemon juice over the tuna.

Buckwheat pasta salad with artichokes, Parmesan and Parma ham

Preparation time: 10 minutes

Cooking time: -

Ingredients:

- ✓ 60 g buckwheat noodles
- ✓ 50 g canned artichokes (in oil or water), drain and cut into bite-sized pieces
- ✓ 130 g (1) tomato, diced or cut into 8 pieces
- ✓ 1 teaspoon capers
- ✓ 10 g red onion, thinly sliced
- ✓ 1 teaspoon extra virgin olive oil juice
- ✓ Juice of ¼ - ½ lemon, depending on taste
- ✓ 1 tbsp chopped parsley
- ✓ 2 slices of Parma ham or other ham
- ✓ 20 g rocket
- ✓ 15 g parmesan or other hard Italian cheese

Nutritional values: (1 serving)

Carbohydrates: 26 | Fat: 20 | Protein: 8 | Kcal: 330

Preparation:

- • Cook the pasta according to the directions on the package, then drain well and set aside. Mix the artichokes, tomatoes, capers, red onions, olive oil, lemon juice and parsley in a bowl.
- • Mix with the cooked pasta. Cut or tear the ham into 3–4 pieces and mix in the pasta. Place the pasta on top of the rocket, grate the parmesan over it or shave and serve.

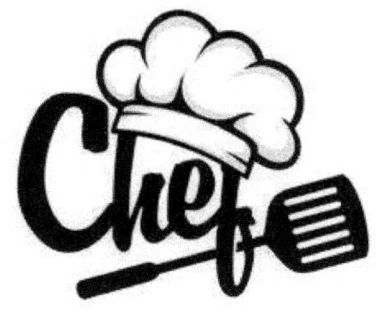

Chicken, Quinoa and Avocado Salad

Preparation time: 15 minutes
Cooking time: -

Ingredients:
- ✓ 50 g quinoa
- ✓ 20 g red onion, thinly sliced
- ✓ 1 teaspoon capers
- ✓ 1 tbsp chopped parsley
- ✓ 20 g sun-dried tomatoes finely chopped
- ✓ 1 teaspoon extra virgin olive oil juice
- ✓ Juice of ¼ - ½ lemon, depending on taste
- ✓ 100 g cooked chicken breast, cut into bite-sized pieces ½ avocado, sliced
- ✓ 20 g rocket

Nutritional values: (1 serving)
Carbohydrates: 22 | Fat: 19 | Protein: 12 | Kcal: 280

Preparation:
- Cook the quinoa as directed on the package, drain well and place in a bowl.
- Mix the onion, capers, parsley, sun-dried tomatoes, olive oil and lemon juice and stir this mixture through the cooked quinoa.
- Add the chicken and avocado to the quinoa mixture and serve on top of the rocket.

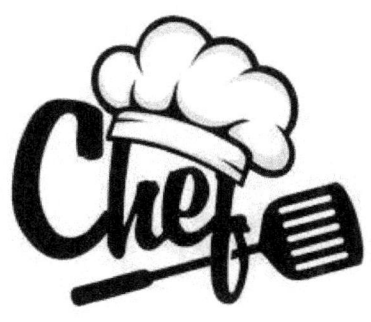

15 minutes Watercress soup

Preparation time: 10 minutes

Cooking time: -

Ingredients:
- ✓ 2 teaspoons of native olive oil
- ✓ 30 g of celery, smaller ties
- ✓ 30 g white onion, smaller rights
- ✓ 200 ml vegetable broth
- ✓ 50 g canned or homemade white beans such as cannellini or haricot
- ✓ 75 g watercress
- ✓ 1 tbsp chopped parsley

Nutritional values: (1 serving)

Carbohydrates: 13 | Fat: 11 | Protein: 5 | Kcal: 130

Preparation:

• Put 1 teaspoon of olive oil in a small saucepan and cook the celery and onion gently for 2 minutes. Add the stock and beans, bring to a boil and cook over medium heat for 10 minutes.

• Chop roughly the watercress and parsley, add to the pan and cook for 1 minute.

• Remove from heat and stir until smooth. Serve the soup drizzled with the remaining teaspoon of olive oil.

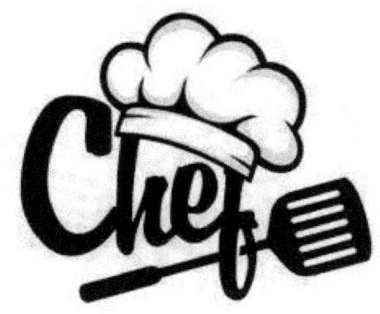

Broccoli beans Artichoke salad

Preparation time: 10 minutes

Cooking time: -

Ingredients:
- ✓ 60 g broccoli florets
- ✓ 75 g tinned or homemade white beans such as cannellini or haricot
- ✓ 20 g red onion, thinly sliced
- ✓ 40 g canned artichokes (in oil or brine), cut into quarters
- ✓ 15 g small black olives
- ✓ 1 tbsp chopped parsley
- ✓ Juice of ¼ - ½ lemon, depending on taste
- ✓ 1 teaspoon extra virgin olive oil
- ✓ 30 g rocket
- ✓ 1 tbsp pumpkin seeds, roasted

Nutritional values: (1 serving)

Carbohydrates: 33 | Fat: 10 | Protein: 7 | Kcal: 310

Preparation:

• Finely chop the broccoli until it roughly resembles the texture of couscous. Alternatively, you can put the broccoli in a food processor for a similar result.

• Mix all remaining ingredients except rocket and pumpkin seeds in a bowl.

• Pour the broccoli mixture on the rocket, sprinkle over the pumpkin seeds and serve.

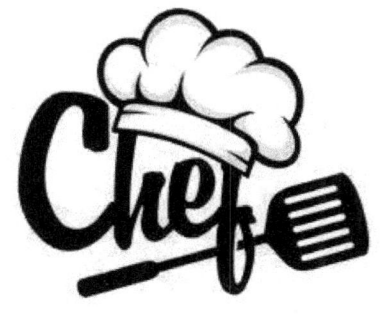

Smoked trout, watercress and potato salad

Preparation time: 15 minutes
Cooking time: 30 minutes

Ingredients:
- ✓ 100 g of new potatoes
- ✓ 1 teaspoon capers
- ✓ 1 teaspoon extra virgin olive oil
- ✓ 1 teaspoon chopped parsley
- ✓ 20 g red onion, thinly sliced
- ✓ 20 g celery, thinly sliced
- ✓ Juice of ¼ - ½ lemon, depending on taste
- ✓ 100 g smoked trout
- ✓ 35 g watercress, roughly chopped

Nutritional values: (1 serving)

Carbohydrates: 8 | Fat: 22 | Protein: 27 | Kcal: 390

Preparation:

• Depending on the size of your potatoes, either cut them in half or cook them in a pan of simmering water for 15 to 20 minutes.
• In a bowl, mix the capers, olive oil, parsley, red onions, celery and lemon juice.
• Drain the potatoes and squeeze them a little with the back of a fork to open them up a little.
• While they're still warm, combine them with the caper mixture.
• Shred or slice the smoked trout and mix with the watercress.
• Serve immediately over the boiled potatoes. If you want, you can squeeze out some lemon juice at the end.

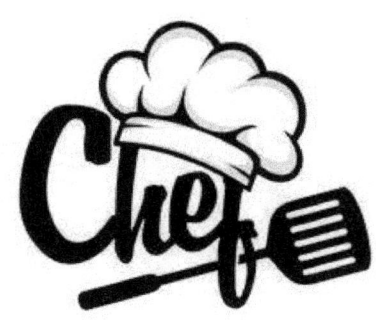

Sirt green bean salad

Preparation time: 15 minutes

Cooking time: -

Ingredients:
- ✓ 20 g red onion, thinly sliced
- ✓ 1 tsp red wine vinegar (or white or apple cider vinegar)
- ✓ 150 g green beans, baked and trimmed
- ✓ 50 g homemade white beans such as cannellini or haricot 4–6 walnut halves, chopped
- ✓ 1 teaspoon capers
- ✓ 100 g tomatoes, diced
- ✓ 2 teaspoons of extra virgin olive oil
- ✓ 1 teaspoon chopped chives
- ✓ 1 teaspoon chopped parsley
- ✓ 25 g rocket and 25 g feta cheese
- ✓ Splash of lemon juice (optional)

Nutritional values: (1 serving)

Carbohydrates: 13 | Fat: 8 | Protein: 5 | Kcal: 130

Preparation:

• Add the chopped onions to the vinegar and set aside to marinate. This will make the onion softer and sweeter. Cook the green beans in boiling water for 4 to 6 minutes, depending on how crispy you like them.

• Drain in a colander and let cool with cold water. Combine the beans, walnuts, capers, tomatoes, oil, and herbs in a bowl then stir in the vinegar and

onion mixture. Serve on the rocket and sprinkle over the feta cheese. Top it off with a pinch of lemon juice if you'd like.

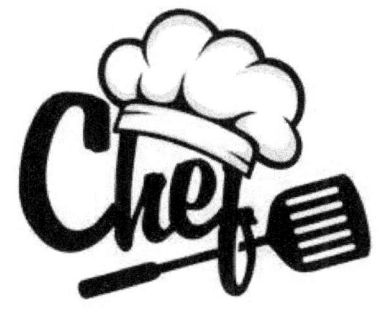

SNACKS

Sirtfood bites

Preparation time: 20 minutes

Cooking time: -

Ingredients:
- ✓ 120 g walnuts
- ✓ 30 g dark chocolate (85 percent cocoa solids), broken into pieces or cocoa nibs
- ✓ 250 g Medjool dates, pitted
- ✓ 1 tbsp cocoa powder (100 percent)
- ✓ 1 tbsp ground turmeric
- ✓ 1 tbsp extra virgin olive oil
- ✓ 1 vanilla pod or 1 teaspoon vanilla extract
- ✓ 1–2 tbsp water (optional)

Nutritional values: (15-20 servings)

Carbohydrates: 20 | Fat: 10 | Protein: 3 | Kcal: 190

Preparation:

• Place the walnuts and chocolate in a food processor and blend until you have a fine powder.

• Add all the other ingredients except the water and mix until the mixture forms a ball. You can add the water if the mixture seems dry, but be careful - you don't want it to be too sticky.

• Shape the mixture into bite-sized balls with your hands and refrigerate in an airtight container for at least 1 hour before eating.

• For a different result, roll some of the balls in more cocoa powder or dried coconut if you'd like.

• The canapes can be stored in the refrigerator for up to a week.

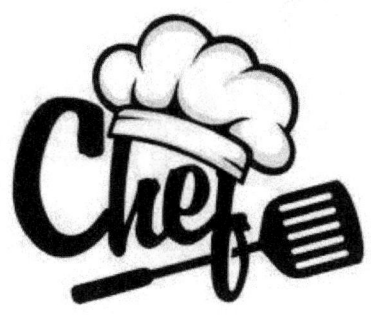

Roasted Cajun Nuts

Preparation time: 10 minutes

Cooking time: 30 minutes

Ingredients:
- ✓ 250 g blanched peanuts or a mixture of pecans, walnuts and hazelnuts
- ✓ 1 tbsp extra virgin olive oil or coconut oil
- ✓ 1 teaspoon paprika
- ✓ 1 teaspoon dried thyme
- ✓ 1 teaspoon sea salt
- ✓ 1 teaspoon oregano
- ✓ 1 teaspoon chili powder

Nutritional values: (2 - 3 servings)

Carbohydrates: 19 | Fat: 11 | Protein: 3 | Kcal: 170

Preparation:

- Heat the oven to 160 ° C / gas 3. Mix all the spices and combine them with the nuts and oil.
- Place the nuts in a single layer on a roasting sheet and sauté for 25-30 minutes.
- Put the roasted nuts in a bowl. After cooling completely, store in an airtight container for up to two days.

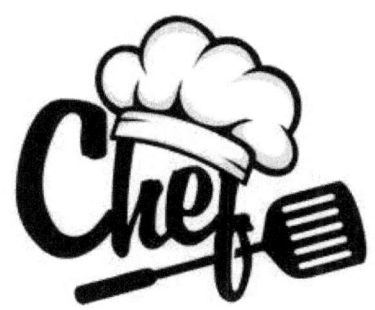

Buckwheat and seed crackers

Preparation time: 10 minutes

Cooking time: approx. 1 hour

Ingredients:
- ✓ 200 g buckwheat flour
- ✓ 50 g sunflower seeds
- ✓ 50 g pumpkin seeds
- ✓ 35 g sesame seeds
- ✓ 1 tbsp extra virgin olive oil + 150 ml water

Nutritional values: *(40 servings)*

Carbohydrates: 11 | Fat: 5 | Protein: 2 | Kcal: 110

Preparation:

• Put all ingredients in a mixing bowl and mix well with your hands. Let rest for 30 minutes, covered with a tea towel or cling film. The mixture may seem a bit runny at first, but the water will be absorbed while the dough rests. Heat the oven to 160 ° C / gas. 3.

• Line a large baking sheet with non-stick parchment paper. Take the dough out of the bowl and shape it into a nice ball with your hands. You may need to add some water if it feels a little dry. Divide the dough in half, place it on a lightly floured work surface and roll it out to a thickness of approx. 1–2 mm.

• You can either bake the dough as individual pieces and then break them or cut into 5–7 cm rounds.

• Roll out any leftover pieces again and stamp out more circles until you have used all of the dough. Repeat for the other half of the dough - you should have around 40 crackers in total.

• Transfer the batter to the lined tray. Bake for 15 to 20 minutes, until light brown and firm. The timing will depend on how crispy you like the finished product. The crackers can be stored in an airtight container for up to 7 days.

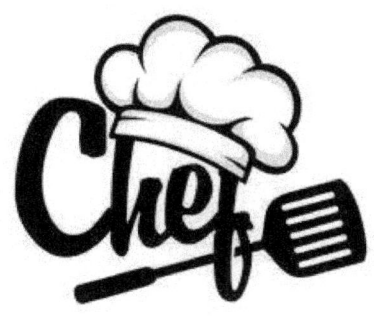

Sea salt and apple cider vinegar Popcorn

Preparation time: 10 minutes

Cooking time: 15 minutes

Ingredients:
- ✓ 50 g corn
- ✓ 1 tbsp extra virgin olive oil
- ✓ 1 tbsp apple cider vinegar
- ✓ 1 teaspoon sea salt

Nutritional values: (2 servings)
Carbohydrates: 14 | Fat: 3 | Protein: 1 | Kcal: 90

Preparation:

• Place a heavy saucepan with a tight-fitting lid over medium heat. Mix the corn and oil, pour the mixture into the hot pan and cover with the lid.

• Shake the pan to get the corn moving in it. Once it starts to pop, turn up the heat and shake the pan for as long as you can while the lid is still on.

• Once the popping has settled down to about 2 to 3 seconds between pops, remove the pan from the heat and empty it into a bowl.

• Discard any unpopped cores. Shake the salt and vinegar over the popcorn and serve warm.

The popcorn can be kept for up to a week in an airtight container.

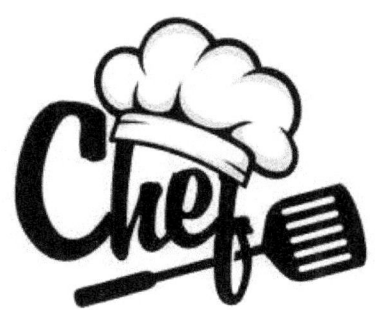

Walnut butter

Preparation time: 10 minutes
Cooking time: -

Ingredients:
- ✓ 350 g walnuts
- ✓ 2 teaspoons of extra virgin olive oil
- ✓ 1 tsp water

Nutritional values: (1 - 2 servings)
Carbohydrates: 7 | Fat: 13 | Protein: 3 | Kcal: 110

Preparation:

- Simply place the walnuts in a food processor and blend for about 2 minutes until you have fine crumbs.
- Gradually add the oil and water and continue until you have a smooth butter. This can be kept for up to 1 week if kept in an airtight container in your refrigerator.

Sirt"Ants on a tree trunk"

Preparation time: 10 minutes
Cooking time: -

Ingredients:
- ✓ 3 stalks of celery
- ✓ 60 g walnut butter
- ✓ 3 Medjool dates, chopped

Nutritional values: (1 serving)
Carbohydrates: 7 | Fat: 5 | Protein: 2 | Kcal: 70

Preparation:

- Cut each stick of celery into three lengths. Using a knife, spread the walnut butter along the central indentation of each piece and place the dates on top.

Peanut energy bar

Preparation time: 10 minutes
Cooking time: 20 minutes
337 calories

Ingredients:
- ✓ 50 g blanched (unsalted) peanuts
- ✓ 200 g jumbo oats
- ✓ 1 lemon peel (washed in hot soapy water first to remove the wax)
- ✓ 50 ml light olive oil and 30 g butter
- ✓ 25 g dark brown sugar
- ✓ 2 heaping tablespoons (50 g) rice malt syrup
- ✓ Juice of ½ lemon 50 g
- ✓ dark chocolate chips

Portioning: (16 servings)

Preparation:
1. Lightly grease a 15 cm square cake pan.
2. Preheat the oven to 160 ° C (140 ° C fan / gas). Mix 2 peanuts, oats and lemon peel in a large bowl.
3. In a small non-stick pan, add olive oil, butter, brown sugar, rice malt syrup, and lemon juice. Heat gently, stirring all the time, until the butter has melted and the ingredients have combined.

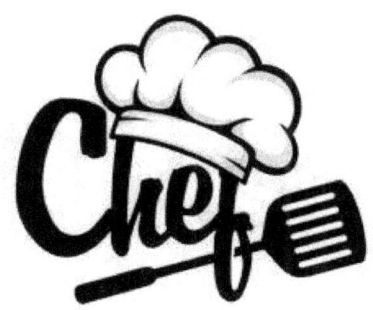

Roasted turmeric nuts

Preparation time: 10 minutes
Cooking time: 20 minutes
195 calories

Ingredients:
- ✓ 250 g blanched peanuts
- ✓ 1 tbsp honey
- ✓ 1 tbsp granulated sugar
- ✓ 1 teaspoon ground cumin
- ✓ 1 teaspoon salt
- ✓ ½ teaspoon chili powder
- ✓ ½ teaspoon ground turmeric
- ✓ ½ teaspoon smoked paprika

Portioning: (8 servings)

Preparation:
1. Preheat the oven to 160 ° C (140 ° C fan / gas 3). Line a baking sheet with a silicone sheet or baking paper.
2. In a large bowl, mix the peanuts with the honey. In a separate small bowl, mix the sugar, cumin, salt, chilli powder, turmeric and smoked paprika together.
3. Add the sugar and spice mixture to the peanuts and toss them well to coat them evenly. Spread the peanuts on the prepared baking sheet. 3 Bake for about 20 minutes, stirring every 5 minutes until the coating begins to thicken. Take out of the oven and let cool down completely

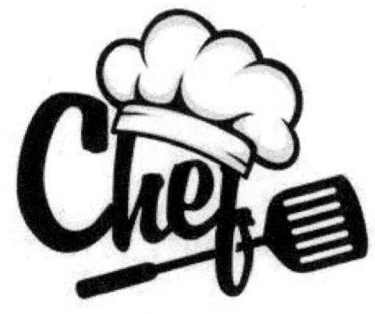

Crispy kale seaweed

Preparation time: 5 minutes
Cooking time: 10 minutes
81 calories

Ingredients:
- ✓ 100 g kale, washed
- ✓ 1 tbsp extra virgin olive oil
- ✓ Freshly ground sea salt
- ✓ black pepper

Portioning: (2 portions)

Preparation:
1. Preheat the oven to 200 ° C (180 ° C fan / gas 6). 2 Remove the tough stalks from the kale and roughly chop them.
2. If necessary, dry the kale on kitchen paper and place it on a large baking
3. sheet.
4. Drizzle with olive oil and sprinkle with plenty of sea salt and a little black pepper.
5. Cook in the oven for 8-10 minutes. Take out of the oven and let cool completely on the tray. Best served on the same day.

Wasabi peas

Preparation time: 10 minutes
Cooking time: 30 minutes
98 calories

Ingredients:
- ✓ 250 g fresh or frozen soy / edamame beans
- ✓ 6 tsp wasabi powder
- ✓ 1 teaspoon salt
- ✓ ¼ teaspoon onion powder
- ✓ 4 teaspoons of water

Portioning: (4 servings)

Preparation:
1. • If you've frozen soybeans, you can thaw them completely on kitchen paper and pat dry.
2. • Preheat the oven to 160 ° C (140 ° C fan / gas 3). Dry the soybeans with kitchen paper before spreading them on a baking sheet and cooking for 30 minutes.
3. • Five minutes before the end of the cooking time, place the wasabi powder, salt and onion powder in a bowl and whisk with the water to make a smooth paste.
4. • Cover and let rest for 5 minutes. When the beans are cooked, take them out of the oven and immediately scoop them into the wasabi paste.
5. • Stir thoroughly to cover all the surfaces of the beans and pour back into the baking sheet to cool and dry.
6. • Leave it in the baking sheet for about an hour before transferring it to an airtight container.

Fried chili tofu

Preparation time: 10 minutes
Cooking time: 20 minutes
132 calories

Ingredients:
- ✓ 150 g firm tofu, cut into cubes
- ✓ 1 clove of garlic, peeled and crushed juice of
- ✓ ½ lemon
- ✓ ½ teaspoon chili flakes
- ✓ ½ teaspoon paprika
- ✓ ½ teaspoon ground turmeric
- ✓ Salt and freshly ground black pepper
- ✓ 1 teaspoon oil

Portioning: (1 portion)

Preparation:
1. Spread the tofu on a plate with kitchen paper. Cover with kitchen paper and set aside to dry.
2. Put the garlic, lemon juice, spices, and a generous spice mixture of salt and pepper in a wide bowl.
3. Mix everything together before adding the tofu and mix gently so that the tofu is completely covered.
4. Let stand for 5 to 15 minutes. Heat the oil in a pan over medium-high heat and wait until the pan is hot before removing the tofu from the marinade and adding it to the pan.
5. Fry for 3–4 minutes, stirring every minute, until the tofu is golden brown all over. Turn off the heat, add the remaining marinade to the pan and serve.

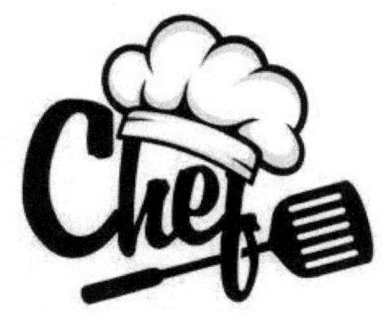

Olive tapenade

Preparation time: 5 minutes
Cooking time: -
132 calories

Ingredients:
- ✓ 1 clove of garlic, peeled and crushed peel and
- ✓ Juice of ½ lemon
- ✓ 1 tbsp capers
- ✓ Drain 3 anchovy fillets, chop them up
- ✓ Drain 200 g pitted green or black olives and roughly chop • 2 tbsp extra virgin olive oil

Portioning: (4 servings)

Preparation:
1. Put the garlic, lemon peel and juice, capers and anchovies in a food processor and stir until smooth.
2. Add the olives and mix again. Do not overmix as some pieces of olive will ensure a good consistency.
3. Scoop out the paste and stir in the olive oil. The tapenade stays in the refrigerator for a few days.

Crispy fried olives

Preparation time: 10 minutes
Cooking time: -
343 calories

Ingredients:
- ✓ 200 g green pitted olives
- ✓ 1 egg, beaten
- ✓ 50 g panko breadcrumbs
- ✓ ½ teaspoon ground turmeric
- ✓ ½ teaspoon paprika
- ✓ 1 tbsp olive oil

Portioning: (2 portions)

Preparation:
1. • Dry the olives on paper towels. Place the beaten eggs in a shallow bowl and mix the breadcrumbs, turmeric, and peppers in another.
2. • Dip and coat the olives in the beaten egg first, then roll in the breadcrumbs.
3. • Heat the oil in a wide pan over medium heat. When hot, add the coated olives and saute until golden brown all over.
4. • Remove with a slotted spoon and drain on kitchen paper before serving.

Turmeric apple chips

Preparation time: 15 minutes
Cooking time: approx. 1 hour
58 calories

Ingredients:
- ✓ Juice of ½ lemon
- ✓ ¼ teaspoon ground turmeric
- ✓ ½ teaspoon ground cinnamon
- ✓ ½ teaspoon ground ginger
- ✓ 1 large apple

Portioning: (1 portion)

Preparation:
1. • Preheat the oven to 120 ° C (100 ° C fan / gas ½). Line two baking sheets with parchment paper or silicone sheets. Put the lemon juice in a small bowl and mix in the spices. Cut off the top of the apple. Using a peeler, cut very thin apple circles across the top. All the seeds in the middle just fall out.
2. • As each very thin slice peeled off, drop it into the lemon juice and lightly mix some lemon juice over it to avoid browning. Discard the base of the apple. Arrange the apple rings in a layer over the baking sheets.
3. • Bake for 1 hour 15 minutes, turn after 45 minutes. Take out of the oven and let cool on the baking sheet before storing in an airtight container.

Chocolate treat

Preparation time: 5 minutes
Cooking time: -
68 calories

Ingredients:
- ✓ 2 heaped teaspoons (20 g) high quality cocoa powder
- ✓ 2 tsp (10 g) granulated sugar
- ✓ Some boiling water
- ✓ 60 ml of milk

Portioning: (2 portions)

Preparation:
1. Put the cocoa and sugar in a small jug. Add a little water from the kettle, just enough to make a smooth paste.
2. Pour in the milk one at a time, stirring thoroughly. Pour into two shot glasses and enjoy your chocolate hit straight away.

Frozen chocolate grapes

Preparation time: 15 minutes
Cooking time: -
97 calories

Ingredients:
- ✓ 50 g good quality dark chocolate (70%)
- ✓ 150 g red seedless grapes

Portioning: (4 servings)

Preparation:
1. • Line a baking sheet with a silicone sheet or baking paper. Break the chocolate into small pieces and place in a small heat-resistant bowl.
2. • Heat a small pan of water, simmer gently and place the bowl with the chocolate on it. Make sure the bowl doesn't touch the water.
3. • Heat and stir the chocolate so that it slowly melts, and remove from heat if there are any lumps left.
4. • Keep stirring the chocolate until everything is melted (this will prevent white spots or blooms from appearing on the chocolate).
5. • Dip the grapes one by one in the chocolate so that they are half coated and immediately place them on the baking sheet.
6. • Proceed with all the grapes. Let the chocolate harden at room temperature before putting it in the freezer.
7. • After freezing, the grapes can be placed in a suitable freezer container. • Serve in servings of 10 to 12 grapes at a time, or just reach in and take a
8. few if needed.

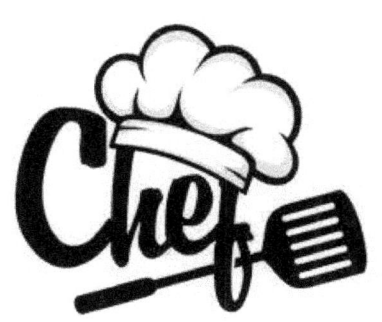

Chocolate Matcha Energy balls

Preparation time: 10 minutes
Cooking time: -
111 calories

Ingredients:
- ✓ 100 g soft dates
- ✓ 100 g blanched almonds
- ✓ 50 g high quality cocoa powder
- ✓ 1 tbsp matcha green tea powder + more to refine
- ✓ 2 tbsp almond milk

Portioning: (10 servings)

Preparation:
1. • Place the dates and almonds in a food processor and process them until they come together into a sticky ball.
2. • Break open the ball with a fork and add cocoa, matcha and almond milk.
3. Mix until they form a large sticky ball.
4. • Take out large, heaping teaspoons of the mixture and roll them into small, tight balls.
5. • Repeat until you have 10 to 12 balls. Dust over a little more matcha powder. These balls stay refrigerated for up to 2 weeks.

DINNER

Beef bourguignon with Mashed potatoes and kale

Preparation time: 15 minutes

Cooking time: 2 - 3 hours

Ingredients:
- ✓ 800 g diced beef
- ✓ 2–3 tbsp buckwheat flour
- ✓ 1 tbsp extra virgin olive oil
- ✓ 150 g red onion, roughly chopped
- ✓ 200 g celery, roughly chopped
- ✓ 100 g carrots, roughly chopped
- ✓ 2–3 cloves of garlic, chopped
- ✓ 375 ml of red wine
- ✓ 2 tbsp tomato puree
- ✓ 750 ml beef broth
- ✓ 2 bay leaves
- ✓ 1 sprig of fresh thyme or 1 tablespoon of dried thyme
- ✓ 75 g diced pancetta or smoked lard
- ✓ 250 g mushrooms
- ✓ 2 tbsp chopped parsley
- ✓ 200 g kale
- ✓ 1 tbsp corn flour or arrowroot (optional)

For the porridge:
- ✓ 500g Edward potatoes
- ✓ 1 tbsp milk and 1 tbsp olive oil

Nutritional values: (4 servings)

Carbohydrates: 34 | Fat: 25 | Protein: 31 | Kcal: 510

Preparation:
- ✓ Pat the beef dry with kitchen paper. Heat a heavy saucepan over medium-high heat. Add the olive oil, then the beef and saute the meat until it is brownednicely all over. Depending on the size of your pan, it's best to do this in 3-4 small loads.

- ✓ When all of the meat is brown, remove it from the pan with a slotted spoon and set aside. In the same pan, add the onion, celery, carrot and garlic and fry over medium heat for 3 to 4 minutes until tender. Add the wine, tomato paste and broth and bring to a boil. Add the browned beef, bay leaves and thyme and reduce the heat to a simmer.

Cover the pan with a lid and cook for 2 hours, stirring from time to time to make sure nothing sticks to the bottom. While the beef is cooking, peel your potatoes and cut them into quarters (or smaller pieces if they're quite large).

✓ Put in a pan with cold water and bring to a boil. Reduce the heat to a simmer and cook for 20-25 minutes, covered with a lid. When soft, drain and mash with olive oil and milk. Keep warm. While the potatoes are boiling, heat a pan over high heat. When it's hot but not smoking, add the diced pancetta.

✓ The fat content of the bacon means you don't need oil to cook it. When some of the fat has been released and it's starting to brown, add the mushrooms and cook over medium heat until both are nicely browned. Depending on the size of your pan, you may need to do this in multiple loads. Set aside after cooking. Cook or steam the kale for 5–10 minutes until soft. Once the beef is tender enough and the sauce has thickened to your liking, add the pancetta, mushrooms, and parsley. If your sauce is still a little runny, you can mix the corn flour or arrowroot with a little water and then stir the paste into the sauce until you have the consistency you want. Cook for 2-3 minutes and serve with porridge and kale.

Turkish fajitas

Preparation time: 15 minutes

Cooking time: approx. 1 hour

Ingredients:

For the filling
- ✓ Cut 500 g turkey breast into strips
- ✓ 1 tablespoon of extra virgin olive oil 1-2 chilies, depending on taste, chopped
- ✓ 150 g red onion, thinly sliced
- ✓ 150 g red pepper, cut into thin strips
- ✓ 2–3 cloves of garlic, chopped
- ✓ 1 tbsp paprika
- ✓ 1 tbsp ground cumin
- ✓ 1 teaspoon chili powder
- ✓ 1 tbsp chopped coriander

For the guacamole
- ✓ 2 ripe avocados, peeled (reserve one of the stones)
- ✓ Juice of 1 lime
- ✓ Pinch of chili powder
- ✓ Pinch of black pepper

For the salsa
- ✓ 1 × 400 g can of chopped tomatoes
- ✓ 20 g red onion, diced
- ✓ 20 g red pepper, deseeded and diced
- ✓ Juice of ½ - 1 lime, depending on the size
- ✓ 1 teaspoon chopped coriander
- ✓ 1 teaspoon capers

For the salad
- ✓ 100 g rocket
- ✓ 3 tomatoes, cut
- ✓ 100 g cucumber, thinly sliced
- ✓ 1 tbsp extra virgin olive oil juice of ½ lemon

For serving
- ✓ 100 g cheddar cheese
- ✓ 8 grated whole grain tortilla wraps

Nutritional values: (4 servings)
Carbohydrates: 44 | Fat: 21 | Protein: 30 | Kcal: 450

Preparation:

1. Mix the filling ingredients together and set them aside while you prepare the other parts.

2. Put all of the guacamole ingredients in a small food processor and flash until a smooth paste is formed. Alternatively, you can mash them all together with the back of a fork or spoon.

3. Place the reserved avocado stone in the guacamole - it will keep it from turning brown. Mix all the ingredients for the salsa.

4. Put all the salad ingredients in a large bowl. Put your largest pan on high heat until it starts to smoke.

5. Put the turkey filling in the hot pan - you may need to cook it in 2 to 3 loads as overcrowding the pan will create too much moisture and it will start boiling instead of frying.

6. Keep the pan over high heat and keep moving the mixture so the turkey colors nicely but doesn't burn.

7. In a low oven, keep the cooked meat warm. To serve, reheat the tortillas according to the directions in the package, then sprinkle some guacamole over each package.

8. Top with some cheese and some salsa, then stack the turkey mixture in the middle and roll it up like a large cigar. Serve with the salad.

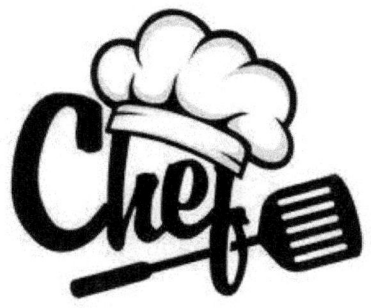

Sirt Chicken Korma

Preparation time: 10 minutes

Cooking time: 50 minutes

Ingredients:
- ✓ 350 ml chicken stock
- ✓ 30 g Medjool date, chopped
- ✓ 2 cinnamon sticks
- ✓ 4–5 cardamom pods, slightly split
- ✓ 250 ml coconut milk
- ✓ 8 boneless, skinless chicken thighs
- ✓ 1 tbsp ground turmeric
- ✓ 200 g buckwheat
- ✓ 150 ml of Greek yogurt
- ✓ 50 g of ground walnuts
- ✓ 2 tbsp chopped coriander

For the curry paste
- ✓ 1 large red onion, quartered
- ✓ 3 cloves of garlic
- ✓ 2 cm piece of fresh ginger
- ✓ 1 tbsp mild curry powder
- ✓ 1 teaspoon ground cumin
- ✓ 1 tbsp ground turmeric
- ✓ 1 tbsp coconut oil

Nutritional values: (4 servings)

Carbohydrates: 21 | Fat: 16 | Protein: 32 | Kcal: 330

Preparation:

1. Put the ingredients for the curry paste in a food processor and flash for about a minute until you have a nice paste.
2. Alternatively, you can grind it with a pestle and mortar. Fry the paste in a heavy pan over medium heat for 1-2 minutes then add the broth, date, cinnamon, cardamom pods, and coconut milk.
3. Bring to a boil then add the chicken legs. Reduce the heat, cover the pan with a lid, and simmer for 45 minutes.
4. In the meantime, bring a pan of water to the boil and stir in the turmeric.
5. Add the buckwheat and cook according to the directions on the package. As soon as the chicken is tender, stir in the yogurt and cook the walnuts over low heat for a few more minutes.

6. Add the coriander and serve with the buckwheat .

Prawns, Pak Choi and broccoli

Preparation time: 15 minutes

Cooking time: 20 minutes

Ingredients:
- ✓ 1 tbsp ground turmeric
- ✓ 400 g raw shrimp, peeled and deveined
- ✓ 1 tbsp coconut oil
- ✓ 280 g buckwheat noodles
- ✓ 1 teaspoon virgin olive oil

For the china pan
- ✓ 1 tbsp coconut oil
- ✓ Cut 250 g broccoli into bite-sized pieces
- ✓ 250 g pak choi, roughly chopped
- ✓ 1 red onion, thinly sliced
- ✓ 2 cm piece of fresh ginger, chopped
- ✓ 1–2 chili peppers, chopped
- ✓ 3 cloves of garlic, chopped
- ✓ 150 ml vegetable broth
- ✓ 1 bunch of basil, removed leaves and chopped stems
- ✓ 1 tbsp Thai fish sauce or tamari

Nutritional values: (4 servings)
Carbohydrates: 13 | Fat: 15 | Protein: 26 | Kcal: 270

Preparation:

• Mix the turmeric with the prawns. Place the coconut oil in a wok or pan and cook the shrimp over medium-high heat for 3 to 4 minutes, or until opaque.

• After cooking, remove from pan and set aside. Wipe the pan for the pan and put it on high heat until it starts to smoke.

• Add the coconut oil then add the vegetables, ginger, chili peppers, and garlic.

• Keep moving the vegetables in the pan so they don't burn. Cook for 3–5 minutes - lower the heat a little if the vegetables look charred - until they are fried but crispy.

• Add the broth, whole basil and fish sauce.

• Bring to the boil, then add the shrimp and let heat. In the meantime, cook the pasta according to the instructions on the package.

• Freshen up in cold water and mix with the olive oil to prevent them from sticking together. Serve the pan with the hot noodles.

Cocoa spaghetti Bolognese

Preparation time: 15 minutes

Cooking time: approx. 1 hour

Ingredients:
- ✓ 1 tbsp virgin olive oil
- ✓ 1 red onion, finely diced
- ✓ 100 g celery, finely diced
- ✓ 100 g carrots, finely diced
- ✓ 3 cloves of garlic, chopped
- ✓ 400 g of lean ground beef
- ✓ 1 tbsp Herbs de Provence
- ✓ 1–2 bay leaves
- ✓ 150 ml red wine
- ✓ 300 ml beef broth
- ✓ 1 tbsp cocoa powder
- ✓ 1 tbsp tomato paste
- ✓ 2 × 400 g cans of chopped tomatoes
- ✓ 280 g whole wheat spaghetti
- ✓ 1 teaspoon ground black pepper
- ✓ 1 bunch of fresh basil
- ✓ 20 g parmesan cheese

Nutritional values: (4 servings)

Carbohydrates: 43 | Fat: 21 | Protein: 11 | Kcal: 450

Preparation:

1. Heat the oil in a pan, then cook the onion, celery, carrot and garlic over medium heat for 1–2 minutes until they are a little softer.
2. • Add the ground beef and dried herbs and cook over medium-high heat until the ground beef is brown.
3. • Add the wine, stock, cocoa powder, tomato paste and canned tomatoes, bring to a boil and simmer for 45 to 60 minutes with the lid closed.
4. • When you're almost done, cook the pasta as directed on the package. • Finally stir the pepper and basil leaves into the sauce. Serve with the
5. pasta and rub some parmesan on top.

Baked salmon with Watercress sauce and Potatoes

Preparation time: 10 minutes

Cooking time: 35 minutes

Ingredients:
- ✓ 400 g of new potatoes
- ✓ 4 × 125 g skinless salmon fillets
- ✓ 1 teaspoon extra virgin olive oil
- ✓ 1 piece of broccoli, cut into florets
- ✓ 1 bunch of asparagus spears

For the watercress sauce
- ✓ 30 g of watercress
- ✓ 5 g parsley
- ✓ 1 tbsp capers
- ✓ 2 tbsp virgin olive oil
- ✓ Extra juice of 1 lemon

Nutritional values: (4 servings)

Carbohydrates: 9 | Fat: 15 | Protein: 31 | Kcal: 250

Preparation:

1. • Heat the oven to 200 ° C / gas. 6. Put the potatoes in a pan with cold
2. water.
3. • Bring to a boil and simmer for 15-20 minutes or until tender.
4. • Brush the salmon fillets with the olive oil, place on a baking sheet and bake in the oven for 10 minutes.
5. • Reduce the cooking time by 2 to 3 minutes if you prefer your salmon to be lightly cooked.
6. • In the meantime, cook or steam the broccoli and asparagus until tender. • Put the ingredients for the sauce in a food processor or blender and stir
7. until smooth. Serve the salmon with the sauce and the vegetables.

Coq au vin with potatoes and green beans

Preparation time: 10 minutes
Cooking time: 35 minutes

Ingredients:

- ✓ 4 skinless chicken legs
- ✓ 4 skinless chicken legs
- ✓ 1-2 tbsp buckwheat flour
- ✓ 1 tbsp extra virgin olive oil
- ✓ 150 g red onion
- ✓ 150 g carrot
- ✓ 200 g celery
- ✓ 3 cloves of garlic, chopped
- ✓ 400 ml red wine
- ✓ 400 ml of chicken broth
- ✓ 1 sprig of fresh thyme
- ✓ 2–3 bay leaves
- ✓ 100 g pancetta or smoked bacon, diced
- ✓ 250 g mushrooms
- ✓ 400 g of new potatoes
- ✓ 2 tbsp chopped parsley
- ✓ 250 g green beans

Nutritional values: (4 servings)

Carbohydrates: 29 | Fat: 16 | Protein: 11 | Kcal: 340

Preparation:

1. • Roll the chicken pieces in the flour. Heat a heavy saucepan over medium-high heat. Add the olive oil then the chicken and cook until nicely browned all over.
2. • Remove from pan and set aside. In the same pan, add the onion, carrot, celery and garlic and cook gently for 2-3 minutes until they soften.
3. • When the pan is dry, you can add some water here. Add the wine and chicken stock and bring to a boil. Add the thyme, bay leaves, and chicken. Cover with a lid and simmer gently for 45 minutes.
4. • Check the amount of fluid from time to time and add a little more. Heat a pan over high heat. When it's hot but not smoking, add the diced pancetta.
5. • When some of the fat has been released and it starts to brown, add the mushrooms and cook over medium heat until both it and the pancetta are nicely browned.
6. • Depending on the size of your pan, you may need to do this in multiple loads. Set aside after cooking.
7. • Put the potatoes in a pan with cold water. Bring to a boil and simmer for 15-20 minutes or until tender. When you're done, drain it and return to the pan to keep it warm.
8. • Add the pancetta, mushrooms and parsley to the Coq au Vin and cook for another 15 minutes.
9. • To cook the green beans, steam them or cook them for 4 to 6 minutes, depending on how crispy you like them.
10. • Serve the Coq au Vin with the potatoes and beans.

Salmon buckwheat Pasta

Preparation time: 10 minutes
Cooking time: 25 minutes

Ingredients:
- ✓ 300 g skinless salmon fillet
- ✓ 1 teaspoon extra virgin olive oil
- ✓ 250 g buckwheat noodles
- ✓ 100 g kale, chopped
- ✓ 1 large zucchini, quarter lengthways
- ✓ Cut 1 red onion into slices
- ✓ Cut 4 cloves of garlic into slices
- ✓ 1 tbsp Herbs of Provence
- ✓ 1 tbsp extra virgin olive oil

For the sauce
- ✓ 650 ml milk or dairy-free alternative
- ✓ 65 g unsalted butter
- ✓ 65 g buckwheat or flour
- ✓ 150 g cheddar cheese, grated
- ✓ 2 tbsp chopped parsley
- ✓ 2 tbsp capers

Nutritional values: (4 servings)

Carbohydrates: 35 | Fat: 13 | Protein: 12 | Kcal: 310

Preparation:
1. • Heat the oven to 200 ° C / gas. 6. Rub the olive oil on the salmon and place it on a piece of foil.
2. • Fold over the edges and seal them to get a package. Bake in the oven for 15 minutes.
3. • Cook the pasta according to the directions on the package. Drain, then pour some warm water out of the kettle to prevent it from sticking and put aside.
4. • To make the sauce, bring the milk to a boil in a small saucepan, being careful not to overflow it.
5. • Then melt the butter in a separate pan and add the flour. Mix them together until you have a mixture.
6. • Cook gently over low heat for 30 seconds to 1 minute. Gradually add the hot milk, stirring continuously, until you have a nice thick sauce.
7. • Add 100 g cheese, parsley and capers and remove from heat.
8. • In the meantime, cook or steam the kale until tender.
9. • In a pan over medium heat, cook the zucchini, red onion, garlic and herbs in the olive oil for 2-3 minutes until tender. Mix with the cooked kale.
10. • Heat a grill on the highest setting. Peel the cooked salmon and mix with the pasta, cooked vegetables and sauce, place in an ovenproof bowl and sprinkle over the remaining cheese.
11. • Place under the hot grill for 5 minutes until the cheese turns brown.

Cauliflower Kale curry

Preparation time: 10 minutes
Cooking time: 30 minutes

Ingredients:
- ✓ 200 g buckwheat
- ✓ 2 tbsp ground turmeric
- ✓ 1 red onion, chopped
- ✓ 3 cloves of garlic, minced
- ✓ 2.5 cm piece of fresh ginger, chopped
- ✓ 1–2 chili peppers, chopped
- ✓ 1 tbsp coconut oil
- ✓ 1 tbsp mild curry powder
- ✓ 1 tbsp ground cumin
- ✓ 2 × 400 g cans of chopped tomatoes
- ✓ 300 ml vegetable broth
- ✓ 200 g kale, roughly chopped
- ✓ 300 g cauliflower, chopped
- ✓ 1 × 400 g can of butter beans, drained
- ✓ 2 tomatoes, cut into wedges
- ✓ 2 tbsp chopped coriander

Nutritional values: (4 servings)
Carbohydrates: 27 | Fat: 17 | Protein: 8 | Kcal: 270

Preparation:

1. • Cook the buckwheat according to the instructions on the package and add 1 tablespoon of turmeric to the water.
2. • In the meantime, cook the onion, garlic, ginger and chili peppers in the coconut oil over medium heat for 2-3 minutes.
3. • Add the seasonings, including the remaining tablespoon of turmeric and continue cooking over low to medium heat for 1–2 minutes.
4. • Add the canned tomatoes and the broth and bring to a boil then simmer for 10 minutes.
5. • Add the kale, cauliflower and butter beans and cook for 10 minutes.
6. • Add the tomato wedges and coriander and cook for another minute.
7. • Then serve them with the buckwheat.

Kidney bean burritos

Preparation time: 15 minutes
Cooking time: 45 minutes

Ingredients:
- ✓ 1 tbsp extra virgin olive oil
- ✓ 1 red onion, diced
- ✓ 3 cloves of garlic, chopped
- ✓ 1 tablespoon chili, chopped
- ✓ 1 tbsp paprika
- ✓ 1 tbsp ground cumin
- ✓ 1 teaspoon chili powder
- ✓ 1 tbsp chopped coriander
- ✓ 2 tomatoes, chopped
- ✓ 3 × 400 g cans of kidney beans, drained
- ✓ 500 ml vegetable broth
- ✓ 150 g cheddar or vegan cheese
- ✓ 8 whole grain tortilla wraps
- ✓ 1 × 500 g glass of tomato passata
- ✓ 1 × 200 g jar of jalepeño peppers (optional)

For the salad:
- ✓ 125 g rocket
- ✓ 1 paprika,
- ✓ 3 tomatoes sliced,
- ✓ ½ small red onion sliced
- ✓ 1 avocado cut into slices, peeled and sliced
- ✓ 1 tablespoon of extra virgin olive oil juice ½ lemon

Nutritional values: (4 servings)

Carbohydrates: 45 | Fat: 24 | Protein: 18 | Kcal: 440

Preparation:
1. • Heat a large saucepan over medium heat. Add the olive oil and sauté the onion, garlic, and chili for 1–2 minutes until a little softer.
2. • Add the spices and coriander and cook for another 1–2 minutes. Add the tomatoes, kidney beans and broth. Bring to a boil and cook over medium-high heat for 20 minutes.
3. • You want most of the liquid to evaporate. So keep an eye on them and stir frequently.
4. • Take off the stove and let cool down a bit. Take about a third of the kidney beans out of the pan and set aside. In a food processor or blender, soften the remaining mixture, then return to the pan, add the whole beans and stir in.

5. • The mixture should be a little stiff. Allowing it to cool completely will make it easier to wrap the burritos. Heat the oven to 200 ° C / gas. 6th
6. • Spread the cheese on top of the wraps, holding back a little to spread over the top at the end. Divide the filling between the wraps and roll each into a sausage tin.
7. • Spread a thin layer of passata on the bottom of an ovenproof bowl large enough to hold all of the burritos in a single layer.
8. • Put them in this way and drizzle the rest of the passata over them. Sprinkle with the remaining cheese and the jalepeños, if used.
9. • Cover the bowl with foil and bake in the oven for 20-25 minutes. Remove the foil and bake for another 5 minutes to brown the cheese.
10. • Throw all the salad ingredients together and serve with the hot burritos.

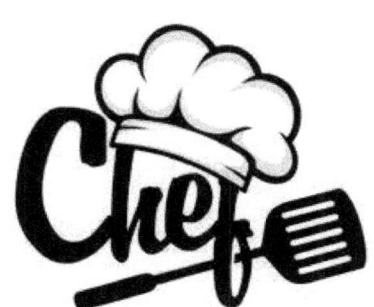

China pan with broccoli, seaweed and Pak Choi

Preparation time: 10 minutes

Cooking time: 15 minutes

Ingredients:
- ✓ 5 g arame
- ✓ 1 tbsp coconut oil
- ✓ 250 g pak choi, roughly chopped
- ✓ 1 red onion, thinly sliced
- ✓ 250 g broccoli, cut into bite-sized pieces
- ✓ 1 large carrot, halved lengthways and sliced
- ✓ 2 cm piece of fresh ginger, finely chopped
- ✓ 1– 2 chilies, finely chopped
- ✓ 3 cloves of garlic, finely chopped
- ✓ 150 ml vegetable broth
- ✓ 1 bunch of basil, leaves removed and stems chopped
- ✓ 1 tbsp tamari (or soy sauce)
- ✓ 100 g cashew nuts
- ✓ 250 g buckwheat noodles
- ✓ 1 teaspoon extra virgin olive oil

Nutritional values: _(4 servings)_
Carbohydrates: 26 | Fat: 16 | Protein: 23 | Kcal: 330

Preparation:

1. • Prepare the arame according to the instructions on the package. Put a wok or large pan on high heat until it begins to smoke.
2. • Add the coconut oil, vegetables, ginger, chili peppers, and garlic. Keep moving the vegetables in the pan so they don't burn. 3-5
3. • Cook for minutes - lower the heat a little if the vegetables look charred - until they are cooked but crispy.
4. • Add the stock, basil, tamari and cashew nuts and let warm for 30 seconds.
5. • In the meantime, cook the pasta according to the instructions on the package.
6. • Freshen up in cold water and mix with the olive oil so that they don't stick together.
7. • Serve the pan with the hot noodles.

Tofu and pumpkin casserole

Preparation time: 15 minutes
Cooking time: 35 minutes

Ingredients:
- ✓ 1 tbsp extra virgin olive oil
- ✓ 1 red onion, diced
- ✓ 100 g celery, diced
- ✓ 100 g carrots, diced
- ✓ 2 cloves of garlic, chopped
- ✓ 1 tbsp Herbs of Provence
- ✓ 1 liter of vegetable stock
- ✓ 2 × 400 g cans of white beans such as cannellini or haricot, drained
- ✓ 1 tbsp tomato paste
- ✓ 500 g butternut squash, cut into bite-sized pieces
- ✓ 100 g kale, chopped
- ✓ 350 g firm tofu, cut into bite-sized pieces
- ✓ 1 tbsp chopped parsley

Nutritional values: (4 servings)
Carbohydrates: 9 | Fat: 20 | Protein: 26 | Kcal: 300

Preparation:

1. • Heat a flame-retardant casserole dish or saucepan over medium heat.
2. • Add the olive oil and sweat the onion, celery, carrot, garlic, and dried herbs for 2-3 minutes until tender.
3. • Add the stock, beans and tomato paste, bring to a boil, then reduce the heat and simmer for 10 minutes.
4. • Add the pumpkin and cook for another 10 minutes. Add the kale and cook for 5-7 minutes or until tender.
5. Add the tofu and parsley, bring to the boil and serve immediately.

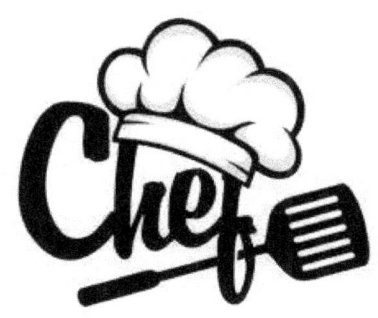

Simple chickpea curry

Preparation time: 10 minutes

Cooking time: 25 minutes

Ingredients:
- ✓ 1 tbsp coconut oil
- ✓ 1 red onion, sliced
- ✓ 3 cloves of garlic, finely chopped
- ✓ 2 cm fresh ginger, finely chopped
- ✓ 1–2 chili peppers, chopped
- ✓ 1 tbsp mild curry powder 1 tbsp ground cumin 2 tbsp ground turmeric
- ✓ 3 vine tomatoes
- ✓ 500 ml vegetable broth
- ✓ 80 g kale, chopped
- ✓ 2 × 400 g cans of chickpeas, drained
- ✓ 2 tbsp chopped coriander
- ✓ 150 ml natural yogurt
- ✓ 300 g buckwheat

Nutritional values: (4 servings)

Carbohydrates: 29 | Fat: 13 | Protein: 9 | Kcal: 360

Preparation:

1. • Heat a large saucepan over medium heat. Add the coconut oil and sauté onion, garlic, ginger and chili peppers for 2-3 minutes.
2. • Add the curry powder, cumin and half of the turmeric and continue cooking over low to medium heat for 1-2 minutes.
3. • Cut each tomato into 8 pieces, making sure to keep as much juice as possible. Put in the pan and cook for 1–2 minutes over medium heat.
4. • Add the stock, kale and chickpeas, bring to a boil and cook for 7–8 minutes over medium heat.
5. • While the curry is cooking, cook your buckwheat as directed on the package, stirring the remaining tablespoon of turmeric into the cooking water.
6. • When the kale is tender, add the coriander and yogurt to the curry, bring to a boil and remove from the heat.
7. • You may want to add a little more water to loosen the sauce. Serve with the buckwheat.

Lentil kale moussaka

Preparation time: 15 minutes

Cooking time: approx. 1 hour

Ingredients:
- ✓ 2 tbsp virgin olive oil
- ✓ 1 red onion, diced
- ✓ 2–3 cloves of garlic, chopped
- ✓ 100 g celery, diced
- ✓ 100 g carrots, diced
- ✓ 1 tbsp oregano
- ✓ 1 tbsp rosemary
- ✓ 2 bay leaves
- ✓ 150 ml red wine
- ✓ 300 ml vegetable broth
- ✓ 1 × 400 g can of green lentils, drained
- ✓ 2 × 400 g cans of chopped tomatoes
- ✓ 150 g kale, chopped
- ✓ 4 large eggplants

For the sauce:
- ✓ 60 g butter or coconut oil
- ✓ 65 g buckwheat flour or flour
- ✓ 750 ml milk or dairy-free alternative
- ✓ 100 g cheddar or similar hard cheese, grated

Nutritional values: *(4 servings)*

Carbohydrates: 21 | Fat: 18 | Protein: 12 | Kcal: 280

Preparation:

1. • In a large heavy-based saucepan, heat 1 tablespoon of olive oil and cook the onion, garlic, celery, and carrot over medium heat for 2-3 minutes until tender. Add herbs, wine and broth and bring to a boil. Add the lentils and tomatoes and bring to a boil, then reduce the heat and simmer for 30 minutes, covered with a lid.
2. • Add the kale and cook for another 10 minutes. In the meantime, heat the oven to 200 ° C / gas. Cut the aubergines lengthways into 1 cm thick slices. Brush the slices with the remaining tablespoon of olive oil and place in the oven on a non-stick tray or on a tray lined with baking paper.
3. • Bake for 7–8 minutes on each side, then transfer to a plate and set aside. Raise the temperature to 220 ° C / gas. 7. To make the sauce, bring the milk to a boil in a small saucepan, being careful not to overflow it.

4. • Then melt the butter in a separate pan and add the flour. Mix everything together until you have a mixture that is neither too runny nor too dry. You may need to add a little more flour or butter to make this happen.

5. • Cook gently over low heat for 30 seconds to 1 minute. Add gradually the hot milk, stirring continuously, until you have a nice thick sauce.

6. • Add all but a handful of cheese, remove from heat, and set aside. To assemble the moussaka, place a small amount of the sauce on the bottom of an ovenproof bowl and distribute it evenly.

7. • Cover with a layer of eggplant, then with the lentil filling, another layer of eggplant, another filling and a final layer of eggplant. Pour the sauce on top and sprinkle over the reserved grated cheese.

8. • Pour the sauce on top and sprinkle over the reserved grated cheese.

9. • Place in the hot oven and bake for 15 to 20 minutes (add 10 to 15 minutes longer if you are warming up from the cold).

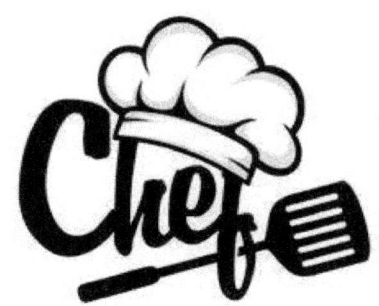

DESSERTS

Vegan vanilla Lemon cheesecake

Preparation time: 10 minutes

Cooking time: 40 minutes

Ingredients:
- ✓ 200 g cashew nuts
- ✓ 160 ml almond, coconut or soy milk
- ✓ 100 g coconut oil
- ✓ 100 g pitted Medjool dates
- ✓ 1 lemon seed from 1 vanilla pod

For the base:
- ✓ 100 g walnuts
- ✓ 75 g pitted Medjool dates, roughly chopped
- ✓ 15 g buckwheat flakes

Optional toppings:
- ✓ 150 g strawberries, chopped
- ✓ 150 g blueberries
- ✓ 150 g vegan dark chocolate (70 percent cocoa solids), grated

Nutritional values: (8 - 12 servings)
Carbohydrates: 55 | Fat: 24 | Protein: 9 | Kcal: 540

Preparation:

1. • Soak the cashews in the milk and set aside while you prepare the base.
2. • For the base, put the walnuts in a food processor and mix to a fine powder.
3. • Add the dates and buckwheat and mix until you have a crumb-like texture. Line the bottom of the tray you have chosen with the crumb mixture and press firmly to form a firm layer.
4. • Put something into the fridge. Put the cashew nuts and their soaking milk, coconut oil and dates in a blender and blend for 2-3 minutes until you get a smooth paste.
5. • Use the finest grater to rub the lemon peel and juice the pulp. Stir them both together with the vanilla seeds into the paste.
6. • Pour the paste over the chilled base (s) and smooth the top with the back of a spoon. Place in the freezer for 2-3 hours until set.
7. • The time depends on the size of your shape. They're a little tough when you serve them straight out of the freezer. So take them out at least 30 minutes before serving.
8. • Add one of the toppings if you'd like.

Date and mocha cups

Preparation time: 15 minutes

Waiting time: approx. 2 hours

Ingredients:
- ✓ 375 ml milk or dairy-free alternative
- ✓ 500 g pitted Medjool dates, chopped
- ✓ Seeds from 1 vanilla pod or 1 teaspoon vanilla extract ½ tbsp strong
- ✓ instant or espresso coffee granulate 2 medium egg yolks
- ✓ 1 tbsp corn flour
- ✓ 100 g dark chocolate (70 percent cocoa solids)

For serving (optional):
- ✓ ½ tbsp cocoa powder (100 percent)
- ✓ Walnut halves, chopped

Nutritional values: (6 servings)

Carbohydrates: 39 | Fat: 21 | Protein: 5 | Kcal: 380

Preparation:

1. • Have six 3-inch casserole dishes ready. Pour 325 ml of the milk into a heavy saucepan. Add the dates and gently heat them, stirring occasionally, to avoid them sticking to the bottom of the pan.
2. • Stir in the vanilla and coffee until the granules have dissolved. In the meantime, mix the egg yolks, cornmeal and the remaining 50 ml milk in a bowl.
3. • Place the chocolate in a heatproof bowl over a pan of boiling water. Be careful not to let the bottom of the bowl touch the water and let it melt. Once it's melted, take it off the stove.
4. • When the milk comes to a boil, immediately remove it from the heat and whisk the cornmeal mixture together. The milk should start thickening immediately. Put the pan back on very low heat and cook for a few minutes until you have a pudding-like consistency.
5. • Pour the pudding over the melted chocolate and whisk until you get a nice shiny finish.
6. • Pour into the baking dishes and let cool before putting them in the refrigerator. Chill for at least 2 hours.
7. • Serve the cups as is, or you can dust them with the cocoa powder or sprinkle them over the roasted walnuts.

Chocolate popcorn cake

Preparation time: 20 minutes

Waiting time: approx. 2 hours

Ingredients:
- ✓ 70 g corn
- ✓ 1 tablespoon of coconut oil
- ✓ 150 g dark chocolate (70 percent cocoa solids)
- ✓ 115 ml milk or dairy-free alternative
- ✓ 55 g pitted Medjool dates, finely chopped
- ✓ 35 g walnuts, finely chopped

<u>Nutritional values:</u> (6 servings)
Carbohydrates: 59 | Fat: 35 | Protein: 11 | Kcal: 600

Preparation:

1. • Place a heavy saucepan with a tight-fitting lid over medium heat. Mix the corn and oil, pour the mixture into the hot pan and cover with the lid.
2. • Shake the pan to get the corn moving in it. Once it starts to pop, turn up the heat and shake the pan for as long as you can while the lid is still on.
3. • Once the popping has settled down to about 2 to 3 seconds between pops, remove the pan from the heat and empty it into a bowl.
4. • Discard kernels that have not been popped and let cool. Place the chocolate in a heatproof bowl over a pan of boiling water.
5. • Be careful not to let the bottom of the bowl touch the water and let it melt. Once it's melted, take it off the heat and gradually beat in the milk until you have a nice shiny ganache.
6. • Stir the dates and walnuts into the chocolate, mix thoroughly, otherwise the dates will clump together.
7. • When the popcorn has cooled, mix it through the chocolate with a spatula, being careful not to overwork it.
8. • Place in cupcake cases and refrigerate for 1½ - 2 hours before serving.

Sirt date pudding with toffee sauce

Preparation time: 25 minutes

Cooking time: -

Ingredients:
- ✓ 250 g pitted Medjool dates
- ✓ 2 tsp bicarbonate soda
- ✓ 200 g of ground walnuts
- ✓ 50 g buckwheat flour, sifted
- ✓ 100 g unsalted butter or coconut oil plus a little more for greasing

For the toffee sauce
- ✓ 200 ml coconut cream
- ✓ 100 g pitted Medjool dates 150 ml water
- ✓ 75 g unsalted butter or coconut oil

Nutritional values: (4 - 6 servings)
Carbohydrates: 29 | Fat: 14 | Protein: 6 | Kcal: 220

Preparation:

1. • Preheat the oven to 170°C / gas 3½. Lightly grease a 20 cm square baking pan. For the pudding, pour 200 ml of boiling water over the dates and let them soak for 5–10 minutes.
2. • After soaking, place the dates and their soaking liquid in a food processor and mix 7–8 times or until you have a coarse paste.
3. • Add the bicarbonate of soda and mix again. Add the ground walnuts, flour, and butter. Flash until you have a nice, smooth paste.
4. • Scoop the mixture into the prepared pan and flatten the lid, then put it in the oven and bake for 30 minutes. (If you prick the center with a wooden skewer, it should come out clean.)
5. • While the cake is baking, make your sauce. Put all ingredients in a small saucepan and bring to a boil. Remove from heat and set aside for 5–10 minutes to cool a little then mix to a smooth sauce.
6. • Depending on the brand of coconut cream you are using, you may need to add some water if it is too thick.
7. • Once the pudding is ready, return the sauce to the saucepan to warm and serve over the warm pudding.

Buckwheat Chocolate chip cookies

Preparation time: 15 minutes

Cooking time: 20 minutes

Ingredients:
- ✓ 120 g dark chocolate (70 percent cocoa solids)
- ✓ Plus 75 g cocoa nibs
- ✓ 20 g cocoa powder
- ✓ 125 g buckwheat flour
- ✓ 1 tsp bicarbonate soda
- ✓ 100 g unsalted butter at room temperature
- ✓ 2 medium eggs
- ✓ 2 tbsp date syrup
- ✓ 1 teaspoon vanilla extract
- ✓ 125 g pitted Medjool dates, finely chopped

Nutritional values: (20 servings)
Carbohydrates: 35 | Fat: 20 | Protein: 3 | Kcal: 380

Preparation:

1. Place the 120 g chocolate in a heat-resistant bowl over a pan of boiling water. Be careful not to let the bottom of the bowl touch the water and let it melt.
2. When melted, remove from heat and set aside. Sift the cocoa powder and flour into a bowl then add the bicarbonate of soda.
3. Using a stand mixer or your fingers, mix or rub the butter into the flour mixture. When you have an even consistency, add the eggs, syrup and vanilla extract and mix well.
4. Stir in melted chocolate, dates, and chocolate chips. Place a 50–60 cm long sheet on your work surface. Put the chocolate mixture in the center and spread it out so that it is elongated.
5. Roll the mixture with the cling film into a sausage form with a diameter of about 4 to 5 cm. As you roll, rotate the ends of the film to get a firm shape.
6. Once you have a tight cylinder, refrigerate the dough for 1 hour. Alternatively, if you find this easier, you can pour the mixture directly onto a baking sheet lined with shortening, in rounds 4–5 cm long.
7. • Preheat the oven to 170ºC / gas 3½. After cooling, cut the rolled dough into 1 cm thick slices and place on a tray lined with baking paper.
8. Bake the cookies for 8 minutes. Let cool on the tray for 5 minutes and then place on a rack to cool completely.
9. • Any mixture that you don't use can be stored in the freezer for up to 3 months as long as it's properly wrapped in cling film.

Quick strawberry mousse

Preparation time: 20 minutes

Cooking time: -

Ingredients:
- ✓ 500 g strawberries, peeled
- ✓ 200 g (2 medium-sized) bananas
- ✓ 100 g Greek yogurt
- ✓ Cocoa nibs at the end (optional)

Nutritional values: (4 servings)

Carbohydrates: 44 | Fat: 21 | Protein: 5 | Kcal: 420

Preparation:
1. • Put all ingredients except the cocoa nibs in a blender and stir until smooth. Transfer to bowls or casserole dishes and serve immediately or refrigerate until ready to use.
2. • Sprinkle some cocoa nibs on top if you want.

Strawberries with Chocolateglaze

Preparation time: 15 minutes

Waiting time: 1 hour

Ingredients:
- ✓ 70 g dark chocolate (85 percent cocoa solids)
- ✓ ½ teaspoon vanilla extract
- ✓ 20 strawberries

Nutritional values: (4 servings)

Carbohydrates: 31 | Fat: 16 | Protein: 3 | Kcal: 310

Preparation:

1. • Place the chocolate in a heatproof bowl over a pan of boiling water. Be careful not to let the bottom of the bowl touch the water and let it melt.
2. • Add the vanilla extract and stir gently. Then take it off the stove.
3. • Line a baking sheet with parchment paper. Dip the strawberries in the melted chocolate, place them on the paper and refrigerate for 1 hour before serving.

Hot chocolate pots

Preparation time: 15 minutes

Cooking time: 20 minutes

Ingredients:
- ✓ 5 g butter or coconut oil for greasing
- ✓ 100 g dark chocolate (70% cocoa solids)
- ✓ 50 ml date syrup
- ✓ 125 g butter or coconut oil
- ✓ 4 medium-sized eggs, separated
- ✓ 50 g cocoa powder (100%)
- ✓ Pinch of sea salt
- ✓ 1 tbsp cocoa nibs

Nutritional values: (4 - 6 servings)

Carbohydrates: 21 | Fat: 18 | Protein: 5 | Kcal: 260

Preparation:

1. • Preheat your oven to 180 ° C / gas 4. Lightly grease four or six 6 cm casserole dishes (depending on how deep you want your pudding).
2. • Place the chocolate, syrup, and butter in a heat-resistant bowl over a pan of simmering water.
3. • Be careful not to let the bottom of the bowl touch the water and let it melt. After combining, remove from heat and set aside to cool.
4. • In a stand mixer or whisk, whisk the egg yolks at high speed until they are twice the size and turn a creamy color. Sift the cocoa powder and salt and mix at a slower speed until well blended.
5. • In a separate bowl, whisk the egg whites at high speed until they form soft peaks - you don't want them to be firm. Carefully fold the egg yolk mixture into the chocolate.
6. • Fold in about a third of the egg white to dissolve the chocolate mixture and carefully fold in the rest. You want to keep the air bubbles in the egg whites as this will make the mixture rise.
7. • Spoon the mixture into the casserole dishes or use a piping bag. Carefully transfer the mixture into the bag and guide it into the casserole dishes, leaving a 1 cm gap at the top.
8. • Use the back of a spoon to level it out then sprinkle with the cocoa nibs. • Bake for 10–12 minutes. They should have risen nicely and cooked on
9. the outside, but melted in the middle.

BEVERAGES

Pak Choi and Rucola green juice

Preparation time: 10 minutes
Cooking time: -

Ingredients:
- ✓ 1 medium (100 g) pak choi
- ✓ a large handful (30 g) of arugula
- ✓ a medium handful (15 grams) of watercress
- ✓ a very small handful (5 g) of chives
- ✓ 2–3 large green celery stalks (150 g),
- ✓ including leaves 1–2 cm piece of fresh ginger Juice of ½ lemon
- ✓ ½ teaspoon matcha

Nutritional values: (1 serving)
Carbohydrates: 15 | Fat: 5 | Protein: 2 | Kcal: 130

Preparation:

1. • Mix the pak choi, arugula, watercress and chives and extract the juice from everything. Now juice the celery and ginger.
2. • You can peel the lemon and put it through the juicer, but it's much easier to just squeeze the juice by hand.
3. • At this point, you should have about 250 ml of juice total, maybe a little more. Only when the juice is made and ready to serve do you add the matcha.
4. • Pour a small amount of the juice into a glass, then add the matcha and stir vigorously with a fork or teaspoon.
5. • Once the matcha has dissolved, add the rest of the juice. Stir it one last time and your juice is ready to drink.

Watercress and lime green juice

Preparation time: 10 minutes

Cooking time: -

Ingredients:
- ✓ 3 large handfuls (75 g) watercress
- ✓ 2–3 large green celery stalks (150 g),
- ✓ including leaves 1 green apple
- ✓ 1–2 cm piece of fresh ginger
- ✓ Juice of 1 lime
- ✓ ½ teaspoon matcha

Nutritional values: (1 serving)

Carbohydrates: 10 | Fat: 8 | Protein: 3 | Kcal: 120

Preparation:

1. • First extract the juice from the watercress, then extract the juice from the
2. celery, apple and ginger. You can peel the lime and also pass it through the juicer.
3. • At this point, you should have about 250 ml of juice total, maybe a little more. Only when the juice is made and ready to serve do you add the matcha.
4. • Pour a small amount of the juice into a glass, then add the matcha and stir vigorously with a fork or teaspoon.
5. • Once the matcha has dissolved, add the rest of the juice. Stir it one last time and your juice is ready to drink.

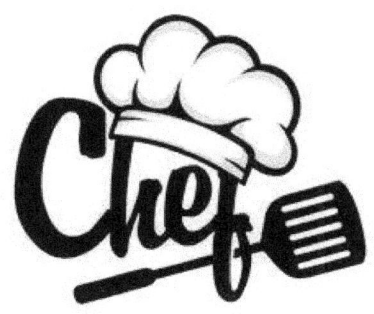

Carrot apple Ginger smoothie

Preparation time: 5 minutes

Cooking time: -

Ingredients:
- ✓ 200 ml of water
- ✓ 25 g carrots, grated
- ✓ 90 g unpeeled apple, sliced
- ✓ 5 g fresh ginger, cut
- ✓ 10 g walnuts
- ✓ 1 pitted Medjool dates
- ✓ ½ - 1 teaspoon ground turmeric,
- ✓ depending on your taste

Nutritional values: (1 serving)

Carbohydrates: 8 | Fat: 3 | Protein: 1 | Kcal: 100

Preparation:

1. • Put all ingredients in a powerful mixer and stir until smooth.
2. • Once the matcha has dissolved, add the rest of the juice. Stir it one last time and your juice is ready to drink.

Berries bananas Smoothie

Preparation time: 5 minutes

Cooking time: -

Ingredients:
- ✓ 150 ml of water
- ✓ 70 g strawberries, peeled and halved
- ✓ 40 g raspberries
- ✓ 40 g blackberries
- ✓ 50 g banana, cut
- ✓ 10 g walnuts

Nutritional values: (1 serving)

Carbohydrates: 6 | Fat: 2 | Protein: 1 | Kcal: 80

Preparation:

1. • Put all ingredients in a powerful mixer and stir until smooth.
2. • Once the matcha has dissolved, add the rest of the juice. Give it one last stir and your juice is ready to drink.

Green tea and Rocket smoothie

Preparation time: 5 minutes

Cooking time: -

Ingredients:
- ✓ 200 ml of water
- ✓ 50 g banana, sliced
- ✓ 25 g pitted Medjool dates
- ✓ 15 g rocket
- ✓ 1 teaspoon matcha
- ✓ 5 g parsley

Nutritional values: (1 serving)

Carbohydrates: 12 | Fat: 5 | Protein: 2 | Kcal: 110

Preparation:
1. • Put all ingredients in a powerful mixer and stir until smooth.
2. • Once the matcha has dissolved, add the rest of the juice .

Chocolate strawberry milk

Preparation time: 5 minutes

Cooking time: -

Ingredients:
- ✓ 150 g strawberries, peeled and halved
- ✓ 1 tbsp cocoa powder (100 percent cocoa)
- ✓ 10 g pitted Medjool dates
- ✓ 10 g walnuts
- ✓ 200 ml milk or dairy-free alternative

Nutritional values: (1 serving)

Carbohydrates: 16 | Fat: 6 | Protein: 3 | Kcal: 130

Preparation:
1. • Put all ingredients in a powerful mixer and stir until smooth.
2. • Once the matcha has dissolved, add the rest of the juice.

Pineapple Lassi

Preparation time: 5 minutes

Cooking time: -

Ingredients:

- ✓ 200 g pineapple, cut into pieces
- ✓ 150 g Greek yogurt
- ✓ 4–5 ice cubes
- ✓ 1 teaspoon ground turmeric

Nutritional values: (1 serving)

Carbohydrates: 13 | Fat: 3 | Protein: 2 | Kcal: 90

Preparation:

1. • Put all ingredients in a powerful mixer and stir until smooth.
2. • Once the matcha has dissolved, add the rest of the juice. If the mixture is too thick, just add some water and mix until you get the consistency you want.

Strawberry Lassi

Preparation time: 5 minutes

Cooking time: -

Ingredients:

- ✓ 150 g strawberries, peeled and halved
- ✓ 150 g Greek yogurt
- ✓ 4–5 ice cubesPinch of ground cardamom

Nutritional values: (1 serving)

Carbohydrates: 11 | Fat: 6 | Protein: 3 | Kcal: 90

Preparation:

1. • Put all ingredients in a powerful mixer and stir until smooth.
2. • Once the matcha has dissolved, add the rest of the juice. If the mixture is too thick, just add some water and mix until you get the consistency you want.

Sirt shot

Preparation time: 5 minutes

Cooking time: -

Ingredients:
- ✓ 3–5 cm (10 g) turmeric root, peeled
- ✓ 4–6 cm (25 g) fresh ginger, peeled
- ✓ ½ medium-sized (70 g) apple, unpeeled
- ✓ Juice of ¼ lemon
- ✓ Pinch of black pepper

Nutritional values: (1 serving)
Carbohydrates: 7 | Fat: 10 | Protein: 2 | Kcal: 110

Preparation:

1. • Put all ingredients in a powerful mixer and stir until smooth.
2. • Once the matcha has dissolved, add the rest of the juice. If the mixture is too thick, just add some water and mix until you get the consistency you want.

Chili chocolate

Preparation time: 5 minutes

Cooking time: -

Ingredients:
- ✓ 1 chili
- ✓ 250 ml milk or non-dairy
- ✓ Alternative 1 teaspoon cocoa powder (100 percent)
- ✓ 35 g dark chocolate (70 percent cocoa solids),
- ✓ 1 teaspoon grated date syrup

Nutritional values: (1 serving)
Carbohydrates: 17 | Fat: 9 | Protein: 4 | Kcal: 150

Preparation:
- ✓ Halve the chilies and cut into 6 or 7 pieces. Place in a small saucepan with the remaining ingredients and bring to the boil over medium to high heat, stirring occasionally, so that the milk does not burn or boil over.
- ✓ • Simmer gently for 2-3 minutes, then remove from heat and let steep for 1 minute. Pass through a fine sieve and serve.

Hot turmeric milk

Preparation time: 10 minutes

Cooking time: -

Ingredients:
- ✓ 275 ml whole milk
- ✓ 1 teaspoon ground turmeric
- ✓ 1 cm fresh ginger, chopped or grated
- ✓ 1 tbsp date syrup
- ✓ Pinch of black pepper

Nutritional values: (1 serving)

Carbohydrates: 18 | Fat: 13 | Protein: 4 | Kcal: 190

Preparation:
1. • Put the milk, turmeric and ginger in a saucepan and bring to the boil over medium to high heat, stirring occasionally, making sure that the milk does not burn or boil over.
2. • Reduce the heat to a simmer and cook very gently for another 5 minutes; This will reduce the bitterness of the turmeric.
3. • Add the date syrup and black pepper and remove from heat. Let it steep for another 5 minutes, cover with a lid, then pass through a fine sieve and serve.

Vegan mocha milk

Preparation time: 10 minutes

Cooking time: -

Ingredients:
- ✓ 250 ml non-dairy milk
- ✓ 50 g vegan dark chocolate (at least 70 percent cocoa solids), grated
- ✓ 1 teaspoon instant coffee granules (or more, depending on how strong you want them)
- ✓ 1 teaspoon date syrup

Nutritional values: (1 serving)

Carbohydrates: 15 | Fat: 7 | Protein: 5 | Kcal: 110

Preparation:
1. • Put all ingredients in a saucepan and bring to the boil over medium to high heat, stirring occasionally, making sure that the milk does not burn or boil over.
2. • Bring to a boil and serve once all of the chocolate has melted.

DRESSING RECIPE

Arugula capers salad dressing

Preparation time: 10 minutes
Cooking time: -

Ingredients:
- 100 ml of extra virgin olive oil
- ✓ 30 ml white wine vinegar
- ✓ 20 ml lemon juice
- ✓ 1 teaspoon capers
- ✓ 1 teaspoon chopped parsley
- ✓ 5 g chopped arugula

Nutritional values: (1 serving)

Carbohydrates: 11 | Fat: 3 | Protein: 1 | Kcal: 70

Preparation:
1. Put all the ingredients in a bowl and mix with a hand blender for about a minute. After emulsifying, transfer to an airtight container and store in the refrigerator.

Chili turmeric salad dressing

Preparation time: 10 minutes
Cooking time: -

Ingredients:
- ✓ 20 g red onion, thinly sliced
- ✓ 1 tsp red wine vinegar (or white or apple cider vinegar)
- ✓ 150 g green beans, baked and trimmed
- ✓ 50 g homemade white beans such as cannellini or haricot 4–6 walnut halves,
- ✓ Chopped
- ✓ 1 teaspoon capers
- ✓ 100 g tomatoes, diced
- ✓ 2 teaspoons of extra virgin olive oil
- ✓ 1 teaspoon chopped chives
- ✓ 1 teaspoon chopped parsley
- ✓ 25 g rocket
- ✓ 25 g feta cheese
- ✓ Splash of lemon juice (optional)

Nutritional values: (1 serving)

Carbohydrates: 15 | Fat: 5 | Protein: 2 | Kcal: 90

Preparation:
- ✓ Put all the ingredients in a bowl and mix with a hand blender for about a minute. After emulsifying, transfer to an airtight container and store in the refrigerator.

JUICES & DRINKS

Green juice

Preparation time: 5 minutes
Cooking time: -
206 calories

Ingredients:
- ¼ avocado, pitted, peeled and roughly chopped
- 1 kiwi, peeled, halved
- 100 ml freshly squeezed apple juice
- ½ ripe pear, pitted, peeled and roughly chopped
- 30 g young spinach leaves, stems removed

Portioning: (1 portion)

Preparation:
- Simply put in the juicer or blender and stir smoothly.

Summer watermelon juice

Preparation time: 5 minutes
Cooking time: -
126 calories

Ingredients:
- ½ cucumber, peeled, halved, seeds removed and roughly chopped if desired
- 20 g young kale leaves, stems removed
- 4 mint leaves
- 250 g watermelon pieces

Portioning: (1 portion)

Preparation:
- Simply put in the juicer or blender and stir smoothly.

Grape and melon juice

Preparation time: 5 minutes
Cooking time: -
125 calories

Ingredients:
- ✓ ½ cucumber, peeled, halved, seeds removed and roughly chopped if desired
- ✓ 30 g young spinach leaves, stems removed
- ✓ 100 g red seedless grapes
- ✓ 100 g melon Melon, peeled, pitted and cut into pieces

Portioning: (1 portion)

Preparation:
Stir in a juicer or blender until smooth.

SIRT fruit salad

Preparation time: 10 minutes
Cooking time: -
172 calories

Ingredients:
- ✓ ½ cup of freshly made green tea
- ✓ 1 teaspoon honey
- ✓ 1 orange, halved
- ✓ 1 apple, pitted and roughly chopped
- ✓ 10 red seedless grapes
- ✓ 10 blueberries

Portioning: (1 portion)

Preparation:
- ✓ Stir the honey into half a cup of green tea. After dissolving, add the juice of half an orange.
- ✓ Let cool down. Chop the other half of the orange and place in a bowl along with the chopped apple, grapes and blueberries.
- ✓ Pour over the cooled tea and let it steep for a few minutes before serving.

Green tea smoothie

Preparation time: 5 minutes

Cooking time: -

183 calories

Ingredients:

- 2 ripe bananas
- 250 ml milk
- 2 teaspoons of matcha green tea powder
- ½ teaspoon of vanilla bean paste (no extract) or the seeds from a vanilla pod
- 6 ice cubes
- 2 teaspoons of honey

Portioning: (2 portions)

Preparation:

- Just mix all the ingredients together in a blender and serve in two glasses.

Kale currants Smoothie

Preparation time: 5 minutes
Cooking time: -
86 calories

Ingredients:
- ✓ 2 teaspoons of honey
- ✓ 1 cup of freshly made green tea
- ✓ 10 kale leaves, stems removed
- ✓ 1 ripe banana
- ✓ 40 g black currants, washed and stems removed
- ✓ 6 ice cubes

Portioning: (2 portions)

Preparation:

- ✓ Stir the honey into the warm green tea until it has dissolved. Mix all ingredients in a mixer until smooth.

Blueberry smoothie

Preparation time: 5 minutes
Cooking time: -
160 calories

Ingredients:
- ✓ 1 ripe banana
- ✓ 100 g blueberries
- ✓ 100 g blackberries
- ✓ 2 tbsp natural yogurt
- ✓ 200 ml of milk

Portioning: (2 servings)

Preparation:
- ✓ Mix all ingredients smoothly and serve.

Grasshopper smoothie

Preparation time: 5 minutes
Cooking time: -
130 calories

Ingredients:
- ✓ 2 large handfuls of kale
- ✓ 30 g (a large handful) arugula
- ✓ 5 g (a very small handful) parsley
- ✓ 5 g (a very small handful) lovage leaves (optional)
- ✓ large stalks of green celery, including leaves
- ✓ half a medium green apple
- ✓ half a lemon, juiced
- ✓ Matcha - green tea

Portioning: (1 portion)

Preparation:
1. • Mix together (kale, arugula, parsley and lovage if used) then juice them out. We find that when juicing leafy vegetables, juicers can vary widely in efficiency and you may need to re-juicing the leftovers before you can move on to the other ingredients. The goal is to get around 50 ml of juice.
2. • Now extract the juice from the celery and apple
3. • You can peel the lemon and pass it through the juicer too- at this point, you should have about 250 ml of juice in total, maybe a little more.
4. • Only when the juice is made and ready to serve, add the matcha green tea. Pour a small amount of the juice into a glass, then add the matcha and stir vigorously with a fork or teaspoon
5. • Once the matcha is dissolved, add the rest of the juice. Give it a final stir and your juice is ready to drink. Feel free to refill with clear water depending on your taste.

Power punch Smoothie

Preparation time: 5 minutes
Cooking time: -
160 calories

Ingredients:
- ✓ 100 g organic yogurt from Greece or coconut
- ✓ 6 walnut halves
- ✓ 8-10 strawberries
- ✓ Handful of kale (stems removed)
- ✓ 1 tbsp raw cocoa powder
- ✓ 1 pitted date (Medjool)
- ✓ 1 teaspoon turmeric
- ✓ 1-2mm slice of bird's eye chili
- ✓ 200 ml unsweetened almond milk

Portioning: (2 portions)

Preparation:
- ✓ Mix all ingredients smoothly and serve.

Date protein smoothie

Preparation time: 10 minutes
Cooking time: -
414 calories

Ingredients:
- ✓ 1/2 cup frozen strawberries
- ✓ 3 stalks of celery, s chopped
- ✓ 1 scoop of whey protein powder
- ✓ 1/3 cup of Greek yogurt
- ✓ 2 Medjool dates
- ✓ 1/2 teaspoon of grated fresh ginger
- ✓ 1 tablespoon coconut palm sugar
- ✓ 1 packet of stevia
- ✓ 1 lemon, juiced
- ✓ 1/2 cup of fresh kale
- ✓ 1/2 cup fresh arugula
- ✓ 1/2 cup of green tea

Portioning: (1 portion)

Preparation:
- • Make tea beforehand and let it cool down. Lemon juice, core, and dates in water. Chop all other ingredients. Then put the ingredients in the blender and stir until smooth.

Classic sirt juice

Preparation time: 10 minutes
Cooking time: -
234 calories

Ingredients:
- ✓ 2 handfuls (75 g) kale
- ✓ Handful (30g) arugula
- ✓ 5 g parsley
- ✓ 150 g green celery (2-3 stalks)
- ✓ ½ green apple
- ✓ ½ lemon - juiced
- ✓ ½ teaspoon matcha powder (green tea)

Portioning: (1 portion)

Preparation:
- ✓ Juice ingredients, should have made 250ml (1 cup) once - enough for 1 juice.
- ✓ Add matcha powder, shake or stir to combine and drink.

Go green smoothie

Preparation time: 5 minutes
Cooking time: -
213 calories

Ingredients:

- ✓ 200 ml orange juice
- ✓ ¼ cucumber with skin
- ✓ 1 great property of kale
- ✓ 1 prize cinnamon
- ✓ 1 apple
- ✓ 1 piece of ginger
- ✓ 1 pear

Portioning: (1 portion)

Preparation:
- ✓ Mix all ingredients smoothly and serve.

Juicy smoothie

Preparation time: 10 minutes
Cooking time: -
317 calories

Ingredients:
- ✓ 150 ml of water or coconut water
- ✓ 1 slice of lemon with peel
- ✓ 1 banana
- ✓ 1 large key spinach
- ✓ 1 apple
- ✓ Juice of 1 orange
- ✓ ¼ avocado without stone

Portioning: (1 portion)

Preparation:
- ✓ Mix all ingredients smoothly and serve.

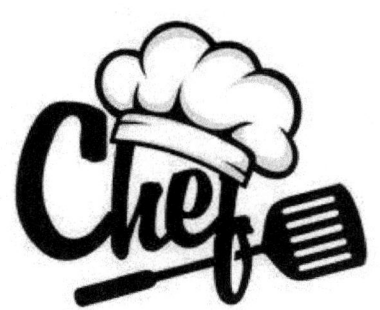

QUICK AND EASY

Spicy bean burgers with spinach salad

Preparation time: 10 minutes
Cooking time: 30 minutes
230 calories

Ingredients:
- ✓ 1 × 400 g cannellini beans, drained
- ✓ 1 tbsp tomato paste
- ✓ 1 tbsp corn flour
- ✓ 2 spring onions, cut and chopped
- ✓ 1 clove of garlic, peeled and chopped
- ✓ 1 teaspoon chili flakes
- ✓ ½ teaspoon ground turmeric
- ✓ Handful (10 g) flat parsley, finely chopped
- ✓ Salt and freshly ground black pepper
- ✓ 1 tbsp olive oil

For the salad:
- ✓ 100 g baby spinach leaves
- ✓ 50 g cucumber, halved lengthways and
- ✓ 2 teaspoons of extra virgin olive oil sliced

Portioning: (2 portions)

Preparation:
1. • Place the beans in a large bowl and mash the beans thoroughly with a potato masher or fork.
2. • Add tomato paste, corn flour, spring onions, garlic, chili flakes, turmeric and parsley. Season generously with salt and pepper. Mix well.
3. • Divide the mixture into four servings and shape them into balls. Then, flatten them a little to form a burger.
4. • If you have time, refrigerate for 20 minutes, or keep refrigerated until needed. The burgers hold their shape a little better when chilled, but are just as tasty when cooked right away.
5. • Heat the oil in a wide pan over medium heat. Put the burgers in the pan and cook for 3-4 minutes.
6. • Turn with a fish slice and flatten it a little more if necessary. Cook for another 3-4 minutes, until golden brown.
7. • Prepare the salad using two serving plates. Spread the spinach and cucumber on both plates.
8. • Drizzle over the olive oil and lemon juice. Serve with two burgers on top and an additional pinch of lemon.

Greek salad skewers

Preparation time: 10 minutes
Cooking time: -
306 calories

Ingredients:

- ✓ 2 wooden skewers soaked in water for 30 minutes before using
- ✓ 8 large black olives
- ✓ 8 cherry tomatoes
- ✓ 1 yellow pepper, cut into 8 squares
- ✓ Cut ½ red onion, halve and cut into 8 pieces
- ✓ Cut 100 g (approx. 10 cm) cucumber, cut into 4 slices and halve
- ✓ 100 g feta, cut into 8 cubes

For the dressing:

- ✓ 1 tbsp extra virgin olive oil juice of ½ lemon
- ✓ 1 teaspoon balsamic vinegar
- ✓ ½ clove of garlic, peeled and chopped
- ✓ Few leaves of basil, finely chopped (or ½ teaspoon dried mixed herbs to replace basil and oregano)
- ✓ 2 teaspoons of lemon juice
- ✓ A few oregano leaves, finely chopped
- ✓ Salt and black pepper

Portioning: (2 portions)

Preparation:

1. • Thread each skewer with the salad ingredients in the order: olive, tomato, yellow pepper, red onion, cucumber, feta, tomato, olive, yellow pepper, red onion, cucumber, feta.
2. • Put all the ingredients for the dressing in a small bowl and mix thoroughly. Pour over the skewers.

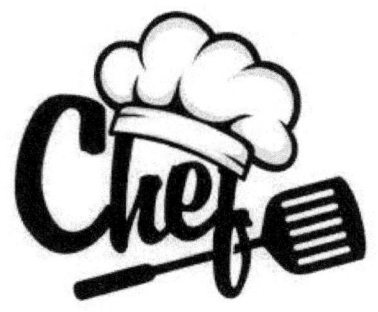

Florentin eggs

Preparation time: 5 minutes
Cooking time: 10 minutes
215 calories

Ingredients:
- ✓ 1 large egg
- ✓ 1 tbsp thick mayonnaise
- ✓ ¼ teaspoon Dijon mustard
- ✓ Juice of ½ lemon
- ✓ 1 teaspoon extra virgin olive oil
- ✓ pinch of salt
- ✓ ¼ teaspoon ground turmeric
- ✓ ¼ teaspoon cayenne pepper
- ✓ 1 teaspoon capers
- ✓ 1 teaspoon (5 g) butter
- ✓ ¼ teaspoon nutmeg
- ✓ 50 g fresh spinach, stalks removed
- ✓ A pinch of paprika

Portioning: (1 portion)

Preparation:
1. • Fill a shallow pot with 4–5 cm of water. Bring to a boil. Crack the egg on the side of the pan and slowly lower it into the water.
2. • Simmer for exactly 1 minute. Turn off the stove and let it simmer in the slowly cooling water for another 9 minutes. This should ensure a boiled egg with a flowing center.
3. • Next, prepare the mock hollandaise. In a small bowl, stir together the mayonnaise, mustard, lemon juice, olive oil, salt, turmeric and cayenne pepper until smooth.
4. • Stir in capers. Heat the butter and nutmeg in a small pan with a lid until the butter just begins to sizzle.
5. • Add the spinach and stir for 30 seconds. Then put the lid on the pan, turn off the heat and let the spinach wither for 2 minutes.
6. • To serve, place the wilted spinach on a small plate, carefully remove the egg from the water with a slotted spoon and place on the spinach.
7. • Pour over the hollandaise sauce and top with a pinch of paprika .

Roast Chicken and Pesto Wrap

Preparation time: 10 minutes
Cooking time: 10 minutes
404 calories

Ingredients:

For the pesto:
- ✓ 50 g rocket leaves
- ✓ 30 g basil leaves
- ✓ ½ clove of garlic, peeled and chopped
- ✓ ½ teaspoon sea salt
- ✓ 50 g pine nuts
- ✓ 20 g parmesan, finely grated
- ✓ 2 tbsp extra virgin olive oil
- ✓ Good pinch of lemon juice

For each wrap:
- ✓ 1 soft tortilla wrap
- ✓ Handful of baby spinach leaves
- ✓ 1 small fried chicken breast fillet (100 g), sliced

Portioning: (4 servings)

Preparation:
1. Put the rocket, basil, garlic and sea salt in a food processor and roughly
2. chop.
3. Add the pine nuts and parmesan and blend again, keeping the pine nuts relatively coarse.
4. Stir in olive oil and lemon juice. Transfer to a suitable container and let the flavors develop.
5. Arrange the spinach leaves for the wrap over the middle third of the tortilla wrap.
6. Add the chicken and pour it over the pesto. Then turn the bottom 2 cm of the wrapping up, pin one edge tightly over the filling, and roll the rest of the wrapping around as tightly as you want.
7. Wrap tightly in cling film and refrigerate until ready to use.

Falafel lunch box

Preparation time: 20 minutes
Cooking time: 15 minutes
387 calories

Ingredients:
For the falafel:
- ✓ 80 g unsalted peeled pistachios
- ✓ 30 g sesame seeds
- ✓ ¼ teaspoon ground cumin
- ✓ ¼ teaspoon ground coriander
- ✓ ¼ teaspoon ground turmeric
- ✓ ½ clove of garlic, peeled and cut
- ✓ 30 g flat parsley
- ✓ Salt and freshly ground black pepper

For the tahini sauce:
- ✓ 2 tbsp (30 g) tahini
- ✓ 1 tbsp white wine vinegar
- ✓ Juice of ½ lemon
- ✓ 2 tbsp extra virgin olive oil
- ✓ ½ clove of garlic, peeled
- ✓ 30 g flat parsley, roughly chopped
- ✓ pinch of salt

For the parsley salad:
- ✓ 150 g couscous
- ✓ Juice of 2 lemons
- ✓ 1 tbsp extra virgin olive oil
- ✓ Salt and freshly ground black pepper
- ✓ ¼ teaspoon ground cinnamon
- ✓ ¼ teaspoon ground coriander
- ✓ Pinch of ground cloves
- ✓ Pinch of ground ginger
- ✓ 4 tomatoes, finely chopped
- ✓ 2 spring onions, finely chopped
- ✓ 50 g flat parsley, stalks discarded, leaves very finely chopped

Portioning: (4 servings)

Preparation:
1. To prepare the falafel balls, simply blend all of the ingredients in a food processor until you have large breadcrumbs. Take heaping teaspoons out of the food processor and shape them into balls by rolling them in your hands. • Set aside or refrigerate in a lidded container until ready to use.

2. For the tahini sauce, put all the ingredients in a mixer and stir until smooth. If necessary, add a little water to dilute it. Set aside or refrigerate in a lidded container until ready to use.
3. For the parsley salad, put the couscous in a bowl and add the lemon juice, olive oil and plenty of salt and pepper.
4. Add all the spices, being careful, especially with the cinnamon and cloves. Stir to mix. Pour enough water over it so that the couscous is generously covered.
5. Let rest for about 10 minutes until all the water is absorbed and the couscous is cooked "al dente".
6. If necessary, top up the water during the rest period. In the meantime, mix the tomatoes, spring onions and parsley together.
7. Mix the salad with the spicy couscous and let the flavors melt together for at least 5 minutes before serving.

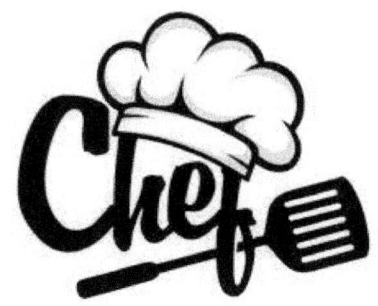

Mexican salsa with cheese and cucumber pittas

Preparation time: 10 minutes
Cooking time: -
324 calories

Ingredients:
- ✓ ¼ red onion, roughly chopped
- ✓ 1 small green chili, cut and pitted
- ✓ 1 spring onion, cut and roughly chopped
- ✓ 1 clove of garlic, peeled
- ✓ 4 large tomatoes, roughly chopped
- ✓ 30g flat parsley
- ✓ ½ teaspoon salt 1 teaspoon olive oil
- ✓ Juice of 1 lime
- ✓ 1 teaspoon tomato paste
- ✓ 1 tbsp water

For each person:
- ✓ 30 g cheese, grated
- ✓ 50 g (5 cm) cucumber, chopped
- ✓ 1 whole grain pitta, quartered

Portioning: (4 servings)

Preparation:
1. • Put the red onion, chili, spring onion and garlic in a food processor and finely chop. Add the tomatoes, parsley, salt, olive oil, lime juice, tomato paste, and water.
2. • Mix until everything is crushed. Transfer to a bowl and let sit for as long as possible so the flavors can pour in.
3. • Mix the cheese and cucumber and spread this on the pittas.
4. • Drizzle or dip the salsa over it if you prefer.

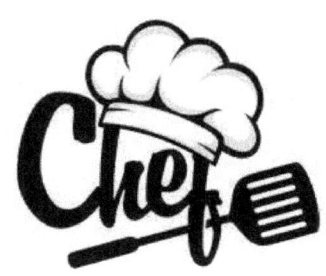

Brie and grape salad lunch box

Preparation time: 5 minutes
Cooking time: -
378 calories

Ingredients:
- ✓ 50 g baby cabbage
- ✓ 50 g (5 cm) cucumber, halved lengthways and sliced Small handful (10 g) of parsley
- ✓ 30 g brie, cut into pieces
- ✓ About 10 red seedless grapes, cut in half
- ✓ 20 g walnuts, halved

For the dressing:
- ✓ 1 teaspoon sesame oil 1
- ✓ Teaspoon extra virgin olive oil
- ✓ Juice of ½ lime
- ✓ ½ teaspoon brown sugar
- ✓ ½ teaspoon salt

Portioning: (1 portion)

Preparation:
1. • Just place the kale, cucumber, and parsley on a serving plate. Spread the brie, grapes and walnuts on top.
2. • Put all the ingredients for the dressing in a small bowl (or a saucepan with a lid) and mix. When you're ready to serve the salad, pour the dressing over it.

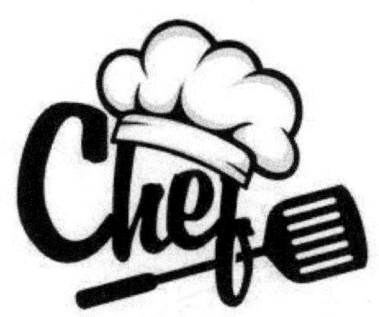

Classic chicken lunch box

Preparation time: 5 minutes
Cooking time: -
272 calories

Ingredients:
- ✓ 50 g fresh or frozen soy or edamame beans
- ✓ 50 g watercress leaves
- ✓ Small handful (10 g) of parsley
- ✓ ¼ red onion, cut into very thin slices
- ✓ 1 small fried chicken breast fillet (100 g), sliced

For the dressing:
- ✓ 2 teaspoons of extra virgin olive oil
- ✓ Juice of ½ lemon
- ✓ pinch of sugar
- ✓ 2 parsley leaves, finely chopped
- ✓ 2 basil leaves, finely chopped
- ✓ 2 leaves of mint, finely chopped
- ✓ Salt and freshly ground black pepper

Portioning: (1 portion)

Preparation:

1. If the soybeans are frozen or need to be cooked, cook them according to the directions in the package and let them cool.
2. Place the watercress, edamame, parsley, and red onion in a serving platter or lunch box container.
3. Add the chicken.
4. Mix the olive oil, lemon juice, sugar, parsley, basil, and mint in a small bowl or container.
5. Season generously with salt and pepper. Drizzle over the salad just before serving.

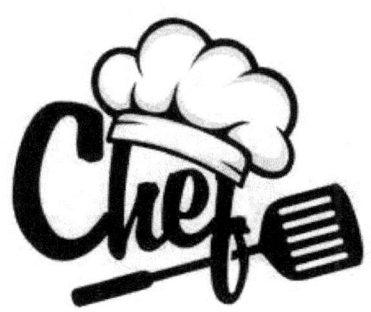

Turkey escalope with sage, capers and parsley as well Cauliflower couscous

Preparation time: 10 minutes
Cooking time: 15 minutes
303 calories

Ingredients:
- ✓ 150 g cauliflower, roughly chopped
- ✓ 1 clove of garlic, finely chopped
- ✓ 40 g red onion, finely chopped
- ✓ 1 chili from a bird's eye view, finely chopped
- ✓ 1 teaspoon fresh ginger, finely chopped
- ✓ 2 tbsp extra virgin olive oil
- ✓ 2 teaspoons of ground turmeric
- ✓ 30 g sun-dried tomatoes, finely chopped
- ✓ 10 g parsley
- ✓ 150 g turkey schnitzel
- ✓ 1 teaspoon dried sage
- ✓ Juice of 1/2 lemon
- ✓ 1 tbsp capers

Portioning: (1 portion)

Preparation:

1. • Place the cauliflower in a food processor and blend in 2-second bursts to finely chop until it resembles couscous. Put aside.
2. • Fry the garlic, red onion, chili and ginger in 1 teaspoon of oil until they are soft but not colored. Add turmeric and cauliflower and cook for 1 minute.
3. • Remove from heat and add the sun-dried tomatoes and half of the parsley.
4. • Brush the turkey schnitzel with the remaining oil and sage and fry for 5-6 minutes, turning regularly.
5. • After boiling, add the lemon juice, remaining parsley, capers and 1 tablespoon of water to the pan to make a sauce then serve.

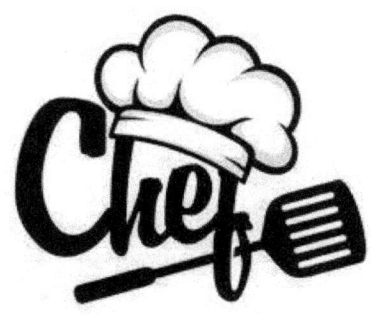

Vietnamese turmeric Fish with herbs & mango sauce

Preparation time: 15 minutes
Cooking time: 30 minutes
294 calories

Ingredients:

Fish:
- ✓ 600 grams of fresh cod, boneless and skinless, cut into wide pieces
- ✓ 2 tbsp coconut oil for frying the fish (plus a few more tablespoons if necessary)
- ✓ Small pinch of sea salt to taste
- ✓ Fish marinade: (Marinate for at least 1 hour or as long as overnight)
- ✓ 1 tbsp turmeric powder
- ✓ 1 teaspoon sea salt
- ✓ 1 tbsp Chinese cooking wine (alt. Dry sherry)
- ✓ 2 teaspoons of chopped ginger
- ✓ 2 tbsp olive oil
- ✓ Infused green onion and dill oil:
- ✓ 2 cups spring onions (cut into long thin shapes)
- ✓ 2 cups of fresh dill
- ✓ Pinch of sea salt to taste.

Mango-dip:
- ✓ 1 medium-sized ripe mango
- ✓ 2 tbsp rice vinegar
- ✓ Juice of ½ lime
- ✓ 1 clove of garlic
- ✓ 1 teaspoon dry red chili (stir in before serving)

Covering:
- ✓ Fresh coriander (as much as you want)
- ✓ Lime juice (as much as you want)
- ✓ Nuts (cashews or pine nuts)

Portioning: (1 portion)

Preparation:
- ✓ Marinate the fish for at least 1 hour.or as long as overnight.
- ✓ Put all ingredients under "Mango Dipping Sauce" in a food processor and mix until you have the desired consistency.

How to fry the fish:
1. Heat 2 tablespoons of coconut oil in a large non-stick pan over high heat. When hot, add the pre-marinated fish. Note: Place the fish slices in the pan one at a time and separate them into two or more batches for frying in the pan if necessary.

2. You should hear a loud hissing sound after which you can turn the heat down to medium high.
3. Don't twist or move the fish until you see a golden brown color on the side (about 5 minutes). Season with a pinch of sea salt. Add more coconut oil to fry the fish in the pan if needed.
4. Once the fish is golden brown, gently turn the fish over to cook it on the other side. Once that's done, transfer it to a large plate.
   Note: There should be some oil left in the pan. We use the rest of the oil to make green onion and dill infused oil.

How to Make the Spring Onion and Dill Infused Oil:
• Use the rest of the oil in the pan over medium heat then add 2 cups of spring onions and 2 cups of dill. Once you've added the spring onions and dill, turn off the heat. Give them a gentle toss until the green onions and dill have wilted for about 15 seconds. Season with a dash of sea salt.
• Pour the spring onion, the dill and the infused oil over the fish and serve with a mango dip sauce with fresh coriander, lime and nuts.

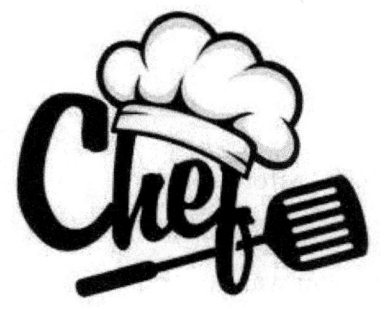

SALADS

French lamb's lettuce

Preparation time: 15 minutes
Cooking time: -
245 calories

Ingredients:

- 1 sprig of mint (5 g), finely chopped
- 1 sprig of basil (5 g), finely chopped
- 1 tbsp extra virgin olive oil
- Juice of 1 lemon
- 1 teaspoon Dijon mustard
- pinch of sugar
- Salt and freshly ground black pepper
- 1 × 400 g cannellini beans, drained
- 1 red onion, drained
- 1 large handful of parsley (20 g) chopped
- 4 tomatoes finely chopped
- ½ cucumber chopped, roughly diced

Portioning: (2 portions)

Preparation:

- Put the chopped mint, basil, olive oil, lemon juice, mustard and sugar in a small amount in the bowl.
- Add a generous spice mixture of salt and pepper. Let rest for 5 minutes. Place the cannellini beans, red onions, parsley, tomatoes, and cucumber in a larger bowl.
- Pour over the dressing and stir. Let rest for 5 minutes before serving.

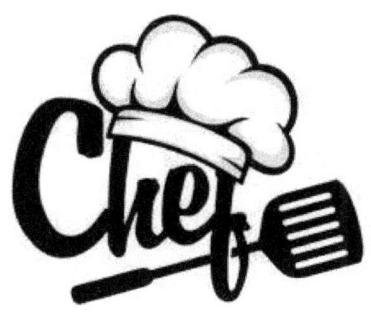

Garlic Butter Chicken Arugula salad

Preparation time: 15 minutes
Cooking time: -
334 calories

Ingredients:
- ✓ 2 cloves of garlic, peeled and chopped
- ✓ 1 tbsp extra virgin olive oil
- ✓ ½ teaspoon dried oregano / mixed herbs Freshly ground black pepper
- ✓ 20 g butter, at room temperature
- ✓ 2 × 150 g skinless chicken breast fillets, cut into strips
- ✓ 80 g rocket leaves
- ✓ ½ red onion, cut very thin strips
- ✓ Large handful (20 g) parsley, roughly chopped
- ✓ ½ cucumber, halved lengthways, pitted with a teaspoon
- ✓ 1 tsp white wine vinegar

Portioning: (2 portions)

Preparation:
- ✓ In a small bowl, combine the garlic, olive oil, dried herbs, and black pepper. Set aside 1 teaspoon of the mixture. Add the butter to the bowl and mix until it becomes a smooth paste.
- ✓ Add the garlic butter to the chicken strips and rub the butter over the chicken pieces with your hands.
- ✓ Set a wide pan on medium heat and mix in the chicken strips when they are hot. Cook for 10-14 minutes, until brown and completely cooked, stirring regularly.
- ✓ Pour the white wine vinegar into the set aside garlic oil and pour over the two salads. Refine with the cooked chicken.

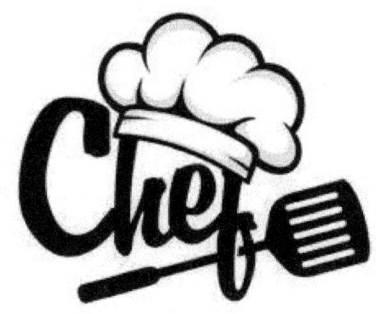

Edamame salad with grilled tofu

Preparation time: 15 minutes
Cooking time: -
293 calories

Ingredients:
- ✓ 200 g firm tofu, thickly sliced
- ✓ 150 g fresh or frozen soy / edamame beans
- ✓ 1 shallot, peeled and very thinly sliced
- ✓ 100 g sprouts
- ✓ ½ cucumber, halved lengthways, pitted with a teaspoon and cut into slices
- ✓ Large handful (20 g) parsley, roughly chopped
- ✓ 1 teaspoon sesame oil salt and freshly ground black pepper

For the dressing:
- ✓ 2 tbsp mirin
- ✓ 2 tsp dark soy sauce
- ✓ Juice of ½ orange
- ✓ ½ teaspoon chili flakes

Portioning: (2 portions)

Preparation:
- ✓ Spread the tofu on a plate with kitchen paper. Cover with kitchen paper and set aside to dry.
- ✓ If the soybeans are frozen or need to be cooked, cook them according to the directions in the package and let them cool.
- ✓ Mix the edamame, shallot, sprouts, cucumber and parsley in a bowl. Mix all the ingredients for the dressing and pour over the salad.
- ✓ Mix everything together well. Heat the grill or frying pan to a high temperature. Brush the tofu with sesame oil on both sides, season generously with salt and pepper and place on the grill tray or frying pan.
- ✓ Cook for 2-3 minutes on each side, turning carefully with a fish slice.
- ✓ Divide the salad on two serving plates and spread the tofu on top.

Baked salmon salad with creamy mint dressing

Preparation time: 20 minutes
Cooking time: -
340 calories

Ingredients:
- ✓ 1 salmon fillet (130 g)
- ✓ 40 g mixed lettuce leaves
- ✓ 40 g young spinach leaves
- ✓ 2 radishes, cut and thinly sliced
- ✓ 5 cm (50 g) cucumber, cut into pieces
- ✓ 2 spring onions, cut and sliced
- ✓ 1 small handful (10 g) parsley, roughly chopped

For the dressing:
- ✓ 1 teaspoon low-fat mayonnaise
- ✓ 1 tbsp natural yogurt
- ✓ 1 tbsp rice vinegar
- ✓ 2 leaves of mint, finely chopped
- ✓ Salt and freshly ground black pepper

Portioning: (1 portion)

Preparation:
- ✓ Preheat the oven to 200 ° C (180 ° C fan / gas).
- ✓ Place the salmon fillet on a baking sheet and bake for 16 to 18 minutes, until just cooked through.
- ✓ Take out of the oven and set aside. If your salmon has skin, simply cook it skin-down and after cooking, remove the salmon from the skin with a slice of fish. It should come off easily when cooked.
- ✓ Mix the mayonnaise, yogurt, rice wine vinegar, mint leaves, and salt and pepper in a small bowl and let stand for at least 5 minutes so that the flavors can develop. 4th
- ✓ Place the lettuce leaves and spinach on a serving plate and top with radishes, cucumber, spring onions and parsley. Put the cooked salmon on the salad and drizzle the dressing over it.

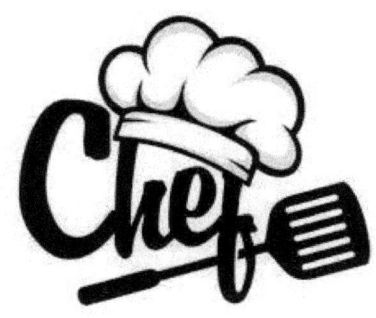

Pomegranate Feta Walnut Salad

Preparation time: 5 minutes
Cooking time: -
390 calories

Allot a **ten:**
- ✓ *75 g young spinach leaves, roughly chopped*
- ✓ *50 g ready-to-eat or cooked Puy lentils*
- ✓ *30 g feta cheese, cut into cubes*
- ✓ *20 g pomegranate seeds*
- ✓ *20 g walnuts, halved*

For the dressing:
- ✓ 1 tbsp Greek style yogurt
- ✓ 1 teaspoon rice vinegar
- ✓ pinch of sugar
- ✓ 1 teaspoon olive oil
- ✓ 2 leaves of mint, finely chopped

Portioning: (1 portion)

Preparation:
- ✓ Combine all the ingredients for the dressing in a small bowl. 2 Place the spinach leaves and lentils on a serving plate.
- ✓ Top with feta, pomegranate and walnuts. Drizzle over the dressing and
- ✓ serve.

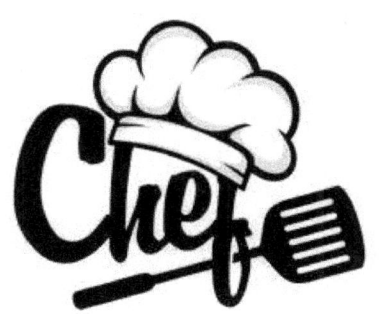

Serrano ham salad

Preparation time: 5 minutes
Cooking time: -
298 calories

Ingredients:
- ✓ 40 g baby cabbage
- ✓ 40 g young spinach leaves
- ✓ Small handful (10 g) parsley, stalks discarded and roughly chopped
- ✓ 2 slices (30 g) Serrano ham, chopped
- ✓ About 12 pitted Kalamata olives, halved
- ✓ Handful (30 g) black currants, washed and stems removed

For the dressing:
- ✓ 1 teaspoon capers, drained
- ✓ 1 teaspoon extra virgin olive oil
- ✓ Juice of ½ lemon
- ✓ Freshly ground black pepper

Preparation:
- ✓ Mix capers, olive oil, lemon juice, and salt and pepper in a small bowl and set aside.
- ✓ Mix the kale, spinach and parsley gently in a bowl. Spread the Serrano ham, olives and black currants on top.
- ✓ Pour over the dressing and serve immediately.

Portioning: (1 portion)

Preparation:
- Mix capers, olive oil, lemon juice, and salt and pepper in a small bowl and set aside.
- Mix the kale, spinach and parsley gently in a bowl. Spread the Serrano ham, olives and black currants on top.
- Pour over the dressing and serve immediately.

Potato salad

Preparation time: 25 minutes
Cooking time: -
348 calories

Ingredients:
- ✓ 120 g new potatoes, quartered
- ✓ 50 g frozen soy / edamame beans
- ✓ 80 g young spinach leaves
- ✓ 40 g smoked salmon, cut into strips

For the dressing:
- ✓ 2 teaspoons of extra virgin olive oil
- ✓ 1 shallot, peeled and very finely chopped
- ✓ 1 teaspoon balsamic vinegar
- ✓ ½ tsp English mustard salt
- ✓ Freshly ground black pepper

Portioning: (1 portion)

Preparation:
- ✓ Steam the new potatoes for 18 to 20 minutes until tender. Add the soybeans for the last 4 minutes of cooking time.
- ✓ Set aside to cool. 2 Very carefully heat the extra virgin olive oil in a small pan. Add the shallot and sauté lightly for 5 minutes.
- ✓ Remove from heat and add balsamic vinegar, mustard, and salt and pepper. Place the spinach leaves over a serving plate. Add the new potatoes and edamame beans. Finally, spread the smoked salmon over it.

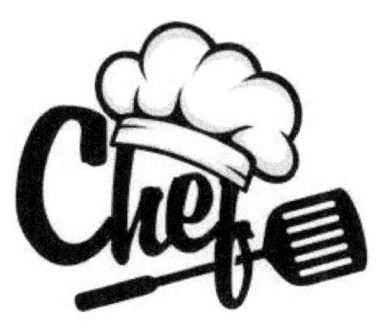

Salad nicoise

Preparation time: 20 minutes
Cooking time: 15 minutes
456 calories

Ingredients:
- ✓ 250 g new potatoes, quartered
- ✓ 50 g fresh or frozen soy / edamame beans
- ✓ 2 large eggs
- ✓ 4 large tomatoes, roughly chopped
- ✓ 10 cm (150 g) cucumber, halved lengthways and sliced
- ✓ ½ red pepper, thinly sliced
- ✓ 50 g high quality black olives, pitted
- ✓ 1 tbsp capers, drained
- ✓ 4 anchovy fillets, thinly sliced
- ✓ Large handful (20 g) parsley, roughly chopped

For the dressing:
- ✓ 1 clove of garlic, peeled
- ✓ 2 anchovies, roughly chopped
- ✓ 3–4 basil leaves salt and freshly ground black pepper
- ✓ 2 tbsp olive oil
- ✓ 1 tsp red wine vinegar

Portioning: (2 portions)

Preparation:
- ✓ Steam the new potatoes for 15 to 20 minutes, until just tender.
- ✓ Add the soybeans for the last 4 minutes if they are frozen or the last minute if they are fresh.
- ✓ Let cool down. 2 Pierce the eggs and put them in a pan with boiling water. Let cook for 9 minutes.
- ✓ Remove and place in a pan of cold water for a few minutes before peeling and quartering.
- ✓ To make the dressing, use a food processor, coffee grinder, or pestle and mortar to grind garlic, anchovies, basil leaves, and salt and pepper.
- ✓ Stir in olive oil and vinegar. Put the tomatoes, cucumber, bell peppers, olives, capers, anchovies and parsley with potatoes and soybeans in a large bowl. Mix gently to mix, add the dressing and mix again.
- ✓ Scatter the quartered eggs on top just before serving .

Sesame Chicken Salad

Preparation time: 10 minutes
Cooking time: 5 minutes
432 calories

Ingredients:
- ✓ 1 tbsp sesame seeds 1 cucumber, peeled, halved lengthways, pitted with a teaspoon
- ✓ 100 g baby cabbage sliced, roughly chopped
- ✓ 60 g pak choi, very finely chopped
- ✓ ½ red onion, very finely chopped
- ✓ Large handful (20 g) parsley, chopped
- ✓ 150 g cooked chicken, shredded

For the dressing:
- ✓ 1 tbsp extra virgin olive oil
- ✓ 1 teaspoon sesame oil
- ✓ Juice of 1 lime
- ✓ 1 tsp clear honey
- ✓ 2 teaspoons of soy sauce

Portioning: (2 portions)

Preparation:
- ✓ Toast the sesame seeds in a dry pan for 2 minutes until they are lightly browned and fragrant. Transfer to a plate to cool.
- ✓ In a small bowl, mix the olive oil, sesame oil, lime juice, honey, and soy sauce to make the dressing.
- ✓ Place the cucumber, kale, pak choi, red onion and parsley in a large bowl and mix gently. Pour over the dressing and mix again.
- ✓ Divide the salad on two plates and top with the chopped chicken.
- ✓ Sprinkle over the sesame seeds just before serving.

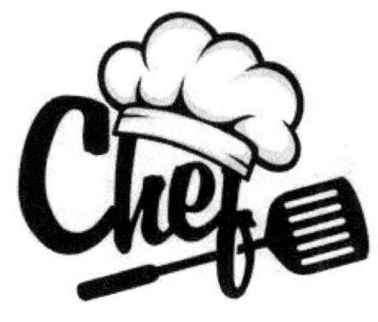

Go-Green Salad

Preparation time: 15 minutes
Cooking time: 5 minutes
304 calories

Ingredients:
- ✓ 100 g small broccoli florets
- ✓ 100 g asparagus, cut
- ✓ 50 g watercress leaves
- ✓ 50 g spinach leaves
- ✓ 200 g ready-to-eat or cooked Puy lentils
- ✓ ½ ripe avocado, peeled and cut into large pieces
- ✓ 20 g pomegranate seeds

For the dressing:
- ✓ 2 teaspoons of extra virgin olive oil
- ✓ ¼ teaspoon ground cumin
- ✓ ¼ teaspoon ground turmeric
- ✓ Juice of 1 lemon
- ✓ 2 tbsp natural yogurt

Portioning: (2 portions)

Preparation:
- Steam the broccoli over a pan of boiling water for 5 minutes or until just tender. Add the asparagus for the last 2-4 minutes (2 minutes for "al dente"). Let cool down.
- Make the dressing by combining the olive oil, cumin, turmeric, lemon peel, and juice with the plain yogurt in a small bowl. Mix the watercress and spinach leaves with the broccoli, asparagus, lentils and avocado.
- Add the dressing and combine gently. Divide between two serving plates and serve with the pomegranate seeds sprinkled on top.

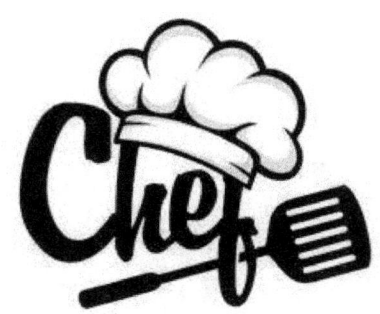

~ 159 ~

Hot chipolata and Currant salad

Preparation time: 15 minutes
Cooking time: 25 minutes
309 calories

Ingredients:
- ✓ 100 g small broccoli florets
- ✓ 1 small shallot, peeled and finely chopped
- ✓ 200 g Chipolata sausages, cut into 2 cm pieces
- ✓ 100 g red currants, frozen and then completely thawed
- ✓ 100 g watercress
- ✓ 100 g young spinach leaves

For the dressing:
- ✓ 1 tbsp olive oil
- ✓ ½ tsp English mustard
- ✓ 1 tsp clear honey
- ✓ 1 teaspoon apple cider vinegar
- ✓ Salt and freshly ground black pepper

Portioning: (2 portions)

Preparation:
- Steam the broccoli over a pan of boiling water for 5 to 6 minutes then set aside to cool.
- Heat a pan over medium heat and add the shallot and chipolatas. Cook for 15–20 minutes, stirring regularly, until the chipolatas are cooked through.
- Turn off the stove and add the red currants. Stir well and let rest in the pan for 5 minutes.
- Make the dressing by mixing together olive oil, mustard, honey, vinegar, and salt and pepper in a small bowl.
- In a large bowl, add the broccoli, watercress, and spinach leaves. Stir half the dressing.
- Divide the salad between two plates, distribute the chipolatas and red currants evenly on the dishes and drizzle over the last dressing.

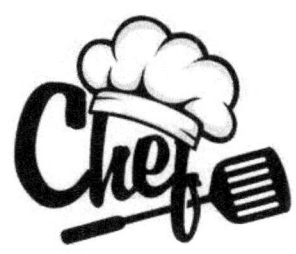

Brie and grape salad with honey dressing

Preparation time: 10 minutes
Cooking time: -
476 calories

Ingredients:
- ✓ 1 lettuce, roughly chopped
- ✓ 30 g rocket
- ✓ ½ cucumber, peeled, halved lengthways
- ✓ 100 g of red seedless grapes cut
- ✓ 1 teaspoon capers cut in half
- ✓ 50 g brie, drained, cut into large pieces
- ✓ 20 g walnuts, halved

For the dressing:
- ✓ 1 teaspoon of liquid honey
- ✓ 2 teaspoons of red wine vinegar
- ✓ 2 teaspoons of virgin olive oil
- ✓ extra pinch of salt

Portioning: (2 portions)

Preparation:
- Put lettuce, rocket, cucumber, grapes and capers in a bowl and mix gently. Mix all ingredients for the dressing in a small bowl and pour over the green salad. Spread the brie and walnuts on top and serve.

Roast Chicken Kale Salad with peanut dressing

Preparation time: 15 minutes
Cooking time: -
383 calories

Ingredients:
- 60 g small broccoli florets
- 150 g cooked and chilled basmati rice
- 60 g kale, chopped
- 60 g young spinach leaves, chopped
- Small handful (10 g) parsley, roughly chopped
- 200 g fried chicken breast, cut
- 10 g sesame seeds

For the dressing:
- 1 heaped teaspoon peanut butter
- 10 g coconut cream dissolved in 30 ml boiling water
- Juice of ½ lime
- ½ teaspoon brown sugar
- ½ teaspoon sesame oil

Portioning: (2 portions)

Preparation:
- Steam the broccoli over a pan of boiling water for 5 minutes or until just ender.
- Put the rice in a large bowl and use a fork to break up any lumps. Add the kale, spinach, broccoli and parsley and stir gently.
- Add the dissolved coconut to the peanut butter one at a time. Stir each time to ensure an even consistency.
- Add the lime juice, brown sugar, and sesame oil. Divide the dressing in half and pour one half over the rice and vegetables and stir.
- Pour the rest of the dressing over the cooked chicken and stir gently until the chicken is completely coated.
- Scoop the dressed chicken over the vegetables and serve with the sesame seeds sprinkled on top.

Smoked trout salad

Preparation time: 20 minutes
Cooking time: -
281 calories

Ingredients:
- ✓ 200 g new potatoes, halved
- ✓ 50 g rocket
- ✓ 50 g young spinach leaves
- ✓ 50 g watercress
- ✓ 8 radishes, cut and quartered
- ✓ Large handful (20 g) parsley, roughly chopped
- ✓ 100 g red seedless grapes, halved
- ✓ 130 g smoked trout, thinly sliced

For the dressing:
- ✓ 1 tbsp mayonnaise
- ✓ 1 tbsp natural yogurt
- ✓ 1 teaspoon olive oil
- ✓ 2 teaspoons capers, chopped
- ✓ 2 cocktail cucumbers, finely chopped

Portioning: (2 portions)

Preparation:
- Steam the new potatoes for 15 to 20 minutes until tender.
- In a large bowl, mix the rocket, spinach, watercress, new potatoes, radishes and parsley.
- Mix mayonnaise, yogurt, olive oil, capers, pickles and lemon juice to make a dressing.
- Stir half of the dressing into the greens.
- Arrange the lettuce and potato on two serving plates. Distribute the grapes and smoked trout evenly on the plates.

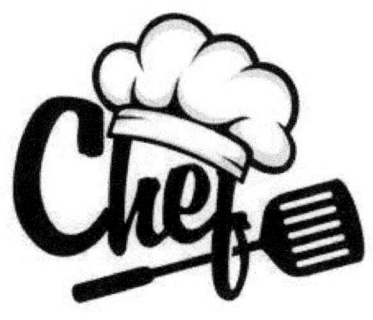

SOUPS

Miso soup

Preparation time: 10 minutes
Cooking time: -
88 calories

Ingredients:
- ✓ 10 g wakame
- ✓ 1 liter of water
- ✓ 5 g (1 sachet) instant dashi granules
- ✓ 100 g tofu, chopped into cubes
- ✓ 1 heaping tablespoon (25 g) white miso paste
- ✓ 2 spring onions, cut and chopped

Portioning: (2 - 3 servings)

Preparation:
- Place the wakame in a small bowl or cup and cover generously with water. Leave on for a few minutes.
- Bring the 1 liter water to a boil in a large saucepan. Stir in the instant dashi powder until it has dissolved.
- Turn the heat to a simmer and add the tofu. Add the wakame to the soup by discarding the water.
- Let simmer for 2 minutes. Put the miso paste in a bowl and add a tablespoon of the dashi broth at a time.
- Stir until the miso has dissolved and you have a smooth, thick sauce. Take the pan off the stove and stir in the miso. Try the soup and add a little more miso if desired.
- Serve in two bowls and sprinkle the chopped green onion evenly over each dish.

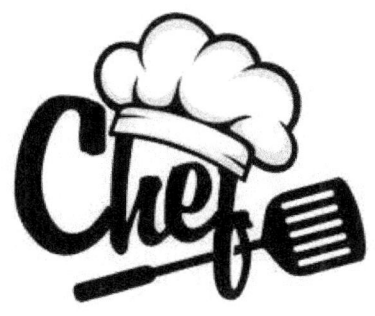

Mexican chicken soup

Preparation time: 10 minutes
Cooking time: approx. 1 hour
361 calories

Ingredients:
- ✓ 4 chicken legs
- ✓ 2 shallots, peeled and roughly chopped
- ✓ 1 carrot, peeled and roughly chopped
- ✓ 1 liter of water
- ✓ 400 g of chopped tomatoes
- ✓ 300 ml passata
- ✓ 1 green pepper, deseeded and chopped
- ✓ 1 red chilli, pitted and finely chopped
- ✓ 2 cloves of garlic, peeled and chopped
- ✓ 1 teaspoon dried mixed herbs
- ✓ 1 teaspoon paprika
- ✓ 1 teaspoon smoked paprika
- ✓ ½ teaspoon ground turmeric
- ✓ ½ teaspoon ground cumin
- ✓ 1 teaspoon mild chili powder
- ✓ 400 g canned black beans, drained
- ✓ 400 g canned kidney beans, drained
- ✓ 30 g (very large handful) parsley, chopped
- ✓ Salt and freshly ground black pepper

Portioning: (4 servings)

Preparation:
- Place the chicken drumsticks, shallots, and carrots in a large saucepan.
- Pour over the water and bring to a boil.
- Cook for 20 minutes, then remove the chicken drumsticks with a slotted spoon and set aside to cool.
- Add the chopped tomatoes, passata, green pepper, chili and garlic and bring them back to boiling point.
- Add the dried herbs, paprika, smoked paprika, turmeric, cumin and chili powder and simmer gently for 30 minutes.
- Remove the skin from the chicken drumsticks and pull as much chicken off the bone as possible.
- Chop the chicken and add it to the pan along with the black beans and kidney beans for the last 5 minutes.
- Remove from heat and stir in the parsley. Season generously with salt and pepper.

Thai spinach soup

Preparation time: 10 minutes
Cooking time: 15 minutes
228 calories

Ingredients:
- ✓ 1 teaspoon olive oil
- ✓ 2 shallots, peeled and chopped
- ✓ ½ teaspoon ground cumin
- ✓ 1 thumb (5 cm) fresh ginger, peeled and grated
- ✓ 1 stick lemongrass
- ✓ 1 red chillies, deseeded, chopped
- ✓ Zest and juice of 1 lime
- ✓ 1 liter of boiling water
- ✓ 400 g coconut milk
- ✓ 250 g fresh spinach
- ✓ 1 tbsp Thai Green Curry Paste
- ✓ Large handful (20 g) parsley, stalks discarded and roughly chopped
- ✓ Large handful (20 g) of coriander, stalks discarded and roughly chopped

Portioning: (4 servings)

Preparation:
- In a large saucepan, heat the olive oil slightly and fry the shallots for 5 minutes until they soften.
- Add the cumin, fresh ginger, lemongrass, chili, and lime zest. Stir thoroughly, then pour in the water.
- Bring to a boil, then add the coconut milk, simmer again slightly and cook for another 10 minutes.
- Add the spinach and curry paste and simmer gently until the spinach is cooked through.
- Remove from heat and throw away the lemongrass stick. Stir in parsley, coriander and lime juice.

Savoy cabbage and bacon soup

Preparation time: 10 minutes
Cooking time: 35 minutes
296 calories

Ingredients:
- ✓ 200 g bacon or pancetta, roughly chopped
- ✓ 2 shallots, peeled and chopped
- ✓ 2 cloves of garlic, peeled and sliced
- ✓ 200 g white potatoes, peeled and roughly chopped
- ✓ 1.2 liters of boiling water
- ✓ 500 ml chicken broth, fresh or made with 1 cube
- ✓ 1 tsp English mustard
- ✓ 800 g savoy cabbage (1 small or ½ large), stalk removed and chopped
- ✓ 200 ml crème fraîche
- ✓ Large handful (30 g) parsley, roughly chopped

Portioning: (6 servings)

Preparation:
- Heat a large saucepan over high heat and toss in the bacon. Fry for 3–5 minutes, turning regularly, until brown and crispy. Remove with a slotted spoon and set aside. Add the shallots, stir and turn the heat on low.
- Let the shallots cook for 5 minutes. Add the garlic and potato, saute them for a few minutes then add the boiling water, chicken broth and mustard. Bring to a boil and simmer for 10 minutes. Add the cabbage, return to the boil and cook for another 6 minutes.
- Put in a blender in two batches and stir until smooth. Put the bacon back in and carefully heat the soup in the pan. Add the crème fraîche with a light fizz and cook for another 2 minutes before serving.

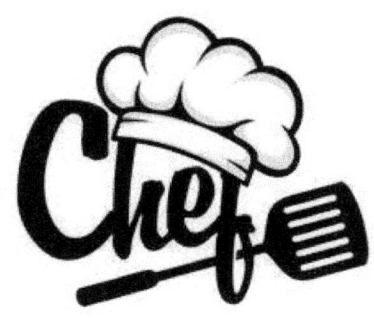

Edamame beans Pesto soup

Preparation time: 10 minutes
Cooking time: 40 minutes
272 calories

Ingredients:
- ✓ 1 teaspoon olive oil
- ✓ 1 leek, cut and sliced
- ✓ 1 clove of garlic, peeled and sliced
- ✓ 100 g white potatoes, peeled and diced 200 g fresh or frozen soy / edamame beans
- ✓ 3-4 basil leaves, torn
- ✓ 750 ml vegetable stock, fresh or prepared
- ✓ 50 g baby leaf spinach, shredded
- ✓ 1 tbsp pesto

Portioning: (2 portions)

Preparation:
- Heat the oil in a large saucepan and gently fry the leek and garlic for 10 minutes. Add the potato, three quarters of the soybeans and the basil.
- Add the broth, bring to a boil and simmer gently for 20 minutes. 2 Put the soup in a blender and stir until smooth. Return the soup to the pan and let it simmer gently. Stir in the remaining soybeans, spinach and pesto and heat for another 5 minutes.

Spicy butternut squash and kale soup

Preparation time: 10 minutes
Cooking time: 20 minutes
340 calories

Ingredients:
- ✓ 1 tbsp olive oil
- ✓ 2 shallots, peeled and chopped
- ✓ 1 clove of garlic, peeled and sliced
- ✓ 200 g sweet potato, peeled and diced
- ✓ 800 g (1 small) butternut squash, pitted, peeled and diced
- ✓ 1 red chili, pitted and chopped
- ✓ 1 teaspoon smoked paprika
- ✓ ½ teaspoon paprika
- ✓ 1 teaspoon ground turmeric
- ✓ 1 teaspoon salt
- ✓ 500 ml vegetable stock, fresh or prepared
- ✓ 1 liter of boiling water
- ✓ 1 tbsp whole grain mustard
- ✓ 20 g parmesan, finely grated
- ✓ 200 g of kale leaves, removed stems and roughly chopped
- ✓ 200 ml crème fraîche

Portioning: (4 servings)

Preparation:
- Heat the oil in a large, thick-bottomed saucepan. Add shallots and garlic and stir-fry for 5 minutes.
- Add the sweet potato and butternut squash. Stir, cover and cook gently for 10 minutes.
- Stir in the chili, paprika, turmeric and salt. Add the stock and water and bring to a boil. Let simmer for 20 minutes.
- Put in a blender in two batches and stir until smooth. Return to the pan and gently heat it.
- Add the mustard, parmesan and kale. Cook for 5 minutes until the kale is tender. Add the

crème fraîche, bring back to temperature and serve.

Kale Stilton Soup

Preparation time: 10 minutes
Cooking time: 30 minutes
232 calories

Ingredients:
- ✓ 1 tbsp olive oil
- ✓ 2 shallots, peeled and diced
- ✓ 2 leeks, cut and sliced
- ✓ 150 g white potatoes, peeled and diced
- ✓ 500 ml vegetable stock, fresh
- ✓ 500 ml of boiling water
- ✓ 400 g kale leaves, stems removed and roughly chopped
- ✓ 2 tbsp (30 ml)
- ✓ Sherry 200 ml skimmed milk
- ✓ 2 tbsp (30 ml) double cream (45% fat)
- ✓ 50 g Stilton, crumbled
- ✓ Large handful (20 g) parsley, roughly chopped
- ✓ Salt and freshly ground black pepper

Portioning: (4 servings)

Preparation:
- Heat the oil in a large saucepan and gently fry the shallots and leeks for 10 minutes until tender.
- Stir in the potato then add the stock and the boiling water. Bring to a boil, then reduce the heat and simmer gently for 15 minutes.
- Use a potato masher to mash the potatoes in the pan - or mix them in a blender if you prefer.
- Add the kale, let it simmer gently, and cook for 4 minutes until the kale is just tender.
- Add the sherry, milk, cream and half of the stilton.
- Let simmer until the stilton has dissolved. Season generously with salt and pepper.
- Divide into four bowls and serve with parsley sprinkled with Stilton.

Curry broth

Preparation time: 10 minutes
Cooking time: 25 minutes
130 calories

Ingredients:
- ✓ 1 tbsp olive oil
- ✓ 2 shallots, peeled and finely chopped
- ✓ 1 clove of garlic, peeled and finely chopped
- ✓ 2 green chilies, pitted and finely chopped
- ✓ 1 teaspoon mild chili powder
- ✓ 1 teaspoon ground turmeric
- ✓ ¼ teaspoon cloves
- ✓ ¼ teaspoon ground cinnamon
- ✓ 1 teaspoon salt
- ✓ 150 g broccoli, cut into small florets
- ✓ 200 g kale leaves, stems removed and roughly chopped
- ✓ 400 ml chicken or vegetable stock, fresh
- ✓ 1 liter of boiling water
- ✓ 250 g tofu, cut into small cubes
- ✓ 2 spring onions, cut and chopped
- ✓ 20 g coriander, chopped

Portioning: (4 servings)

Preparation:
- In a large saucepan with a thick bottom, heat the oil over low heat.
- Add the shallots and saute them for 5 minutes, until they just start to soften.
- Add the garlic, green chilies, spices, and salt. Stir then add the broccoli and kale.
- Fry for 2-3 minutes. Add the stock and water and bring to a boil.
- Let simmer gently for 15 minutes.
- Add the tofu, spring onions, and coriander and cook for a few more minutes until it warms up.

FAST MEALS

Grilled chicken with Lemon and olives

Preparation time: 10 minutes
Cooking time: 40 minutes
270 calories

Ingredients:
- ✓ 2 skinless chicken breast fillets
- ✓ 1 teaspoon olive oil
- ✓ Juice of 1 lemon
- ✓ ½ clove of garlic, peeled and chopped
- ✓ 50 g high quality green olives, pitted and halved
- ✓ 1 tbsp extra virgin olive oil
- ✓ 1 tsp balsamic vinegar
- ✓ Large handful (20 g) parsley, finely chopped
- ✓ Salt and freshly ground black pepper

Portioning: (2 portions)

Preparation:
- Turn the grill on to a medium to high setting.
- Halve the chicken breast. Make another cut in the thickest part of each chicken piece.
- Rub each piece with a little olive oil and place them all on the grill tray. Cook for between 10 and 20 minutes, turning halfway through the cooking process so that the chicken is browned on the outside and cooked through.
- The size of the chicken pieces and the wide variation from grill to grill make it difficult to set an exact time. Obviously, this dish works well in other cooking methods too, including grilling.
- Prepare the marinade in a shallow bowl where the chicken pieces can lay flat. Simply add the lemon zest and juice, garlic, halved olives, extra virgin olive oil, balsamic vinegar, chopped parsley and a generous spice mixture of salt and pepper straight to the serving plate.
- Stir roughly. When the chicken is cooked, immediately put it on the platter, turning each piece so that it is completely covered in the sauce.
- Let rest in the bowl for 2-3 minutes before serving and drizzle the remaining marinade over the chicken as you serve.

Delicious salmon and potato Delicacies

Preparation time: 10 minutes
Cooking time: 15 minutes
407 calories

Ingredients:

4 new potatoes, quartered
1 teaspoon olive oil
125 g cooked salmon
½ teaspoon ground turmeric
½ teaspoon mild chili powder
¼ teaspoon ground cinnamon
Salt and freshly ground black pepper
1 teaspoon capers
40 g rocket leaves
Handful (10 g) parsley, roughly chopped
Juice of ½ lemon

Portioning: (1 portion)

Preparation:

- Steam the new potatoes for 15 to 20 minutes until tender.
- Heat the oil in a pan over medium heat. Add the new potatoes and sauté them for 3–4 minutes, stirring once, until brown.
- Add the salmon, turmeric, chili powder, cinnamon and salt and pepper and fry for another 2 minutes until everything is cooked through.
- Remove from heat and stir in capers, rocket, parsley and lemon juice.
- Serve immediately.

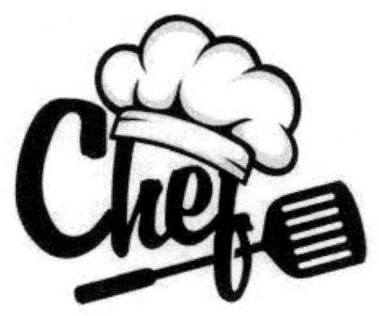

Turmeric prawns

Preparation time: 10 minutes
Cooking time: 10 minutes
414 calories

Ingredients:
- ✓ 1 teaspoon olive oil
- ✓ ½ teaspoon cumin
- ✓ ½ cinnamon stick
- ✓ 2 cloves
- ✓ 1 bay leaf
- ✓ 1 small red onion, chopped
- ✓ 1 red pepper, deseeded and chopped
- ✓ 2 cloves of garlic, peeled and thinly sliced
- ✓ 1 red or green chili, pitted and sliced
- ✓ ½ teaspoon mild chili powder
- ✓ 1 teaspoon paprika
- ✓ 1 teaspoon ground turmeric
- ✓ ½ teaspoon salt
- ✓ 2 fresh tomatoes, roughly chopped
- ✓ 60 g frozen soy / edamame beans
- ✓ 1 tbsp water
- ✓ 250 g cooked king prawns
- ✓ 250 g cooked and chilled basmati rice
- ✓ 50 g rocket

Portioning: (2 portions)

Preparation:
- In a pan with a wide lid, heat the oil over medium heat. Add the cumin, cinnamon stick, cloves, and bay leaf.
- Fry for 1 minute before adding the onion and red pepper. Stir, turn the heat on low and place the lid on the pan.
- Let simmer for 5 minutes. Take the lid off the pan. Add the garlic, chili, chili powder, paprika, turmeric and salt and fry for another minute.
- Add the chopped tomatoes, soybeans, and water. Put the lid back on the pan and cook gently for 7 minutes.
- Take the lid off the pan and remove the cinnamon stick, cloves and bay leaf.
- Add the shrimp and rice and cook for 3-4 minutes until warm.
- Finally stir through the rocket just before serving.

Vegetables with black Bean sauce

Preparation time: 10 minutes
Cooking time: 10 minutes
343 calories

Ingredients:
- ✓ 250 g firm tofu, cut into large cubes
- ✓ 100 g cooked black beans, drained
- ✓ 2 heaped teaspoons (30 g) jam with black currants
- ✓ ½ teaspoon ground ginger
- ✓ 1 tbsp dark soy sauce
- ✓ 1 teaspoon cornmeal salt and freshly ground black pepper
- ✓ 1 tbsp rapeseed oil
- ✓ 1 shallot, peeled and cut into thin slices
- ✓ ¼ Savoy cabbage, stem removed and thinly sliced
- ✓ 100 g kale, stems removed and thinly sliced
- ✓ 1 large carrot, peeled and cut into matches
- ✓ 100 g sprouts cut

Portioning: (2 portions)

Preparation:
- Spread the tofu on a plate with kitchen paper. Cover with kitchen paper and set aside.
- Put the black beans, currant jam, ginger, soy sauce and cornmeal in a food processor and stir until smooth.
- Season the tofu generously with salt and pepper. Heat the oil in a wide pan or in a wok.
- Fry the tofu all around until golden brown over high heat. Remove from pan with a slotted spoon and set aside.
- Add shallot, cabbage, kale and carrot to the pan and stir-fry for 3–4 minutes.
- Add the sprouts and sauté for another 2 minutes. Reduce the heat to medium-low and return the tofu to the pan.
- Add the black bean sauce and warm for 2 minutes before serving.

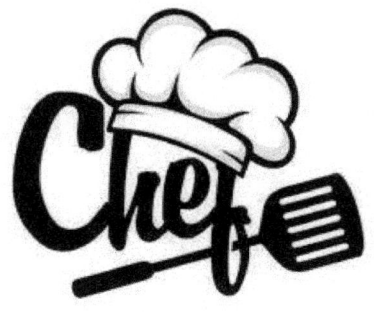

Beef and broccoli

Preparation time: 10 minutes
Cooking time: 15 minutes
409 calories

Ingredients:
- ✓ 1 tbsp corn flour
- ✓ 1 tbsp water
- ✓ 1 clove of garlic, peeled and chopped
- ✓ 250 g roast steak, cut into thin strips
- ✓ 2 teaspoons of rapeseed oil
- ✓ 1 small red onion, cut into wedges
- ✓ 1 small head broccoli, cut into small florets
- ✓ 2 tbsp soy sauce
- ✓ 1 tbsp dark brown sugar
- ✓ ½ teaspoon ground ginger
- ✓ 1 tbsp corn flour

Portioning: (2 portions)

Preparation:
- Mix the corn flour, water and garlic and stir until smooth. Add the steak and stir until thoroughly coated. Heat the oil in a flat, wide pan over high heat. When it's hot, toss in the beef and quickly saute it until fried (or however you want to cook your steak).
- Remove from pan with a slotted spoon and set aside. 2 Add the onion and broccoli to the pan, stir, reduce the heat a little and cook for 4–5 minutes, until they are soft and have a little bite in the broccoli. Mix the soy sauce, brown sugar, ginger and cornmeal together.
- Return the beef to the pan and add the soy sauce mixture. Stir well and cook for another 2 minutes.

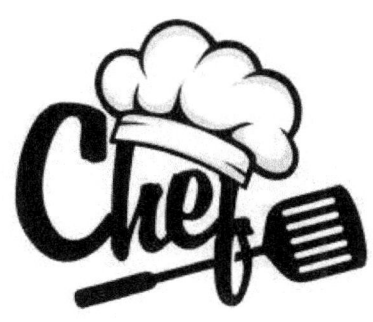

Salmon with soy glaze

Preparation time: 10 minutes
Cooking time: 15 minutes
322 calories

Ingredients:
- ✓ 2 tbsp soy sauce
- ✓ 1 tbsp balsamic vinegar
- ✓ ½ teaspoon chili flakes
- ✓ 1 small thumb (3 cm) fresh ginger, peeled and finely grated
- ✓ 1 tbsp honey
- ✓ ½ clove of garlic, peeled and chopped
- ✓ 2 × 150 g salmon fillets
- ✓ 1 teaspoon olive oil

Portioning: (2 portions)

Preparation:
- Put the soy, balsamic vinegar, chili flakes, ginger, honey and garlic in a wide bowl and whisk with a fork until the honey has dissolved.
- Place the salmon fillets in the bowl skin side up and let sit for 2-3 minutes.
- Heat the oil in a pan over medium to high heat. When it's hot, put the salmon in it but not the marinade and cook it skin up.
- Let simmer for 5–6 minutes. Use a fish slice to flip the salmon so it's skin-down.
- Turn the heat on low. After a minute, pour the remaining marinade around the fish. Let it simmer for another 5 minutes or until the fish is cooked through.
- Serve with the sauce soaked over the fish.

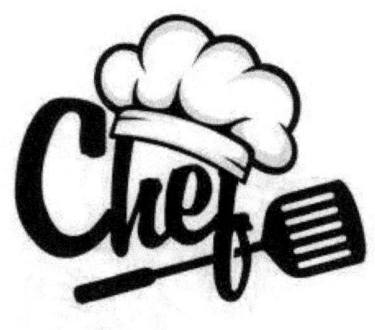

Tandoori spears

Preparation time: 10 minutes
Cooking time: 20 minutes
240 calories

Ingredients:
- ✓ 4 wooden skewers
- ✓ Soaked in water for 30 minutes
- ✓ 400 g firm tofu, cut into large cubes
- ✓ 3 tsp tandoori masala powder (dry tandoori spice mixture)
- ✓ 1 teaspoon of ground turmeric juice from 1 lime
- ✓ Salt and freshly ground black pepper
- ✓ 1 red onion, cut into large slices
- ✓ 1 pepper, deseeded and cut into large pieces
- ✓ 100 g natural yogurt
- ✓ Large amount (20 g) parsley, roughly chopped

Portioning: (2 portions)

Preparation:
- Spread the tofu on a plate with kitchen paper. Cover with kitchen paper and set aside.
- Mix the tandoori masala, turmeric, lime juice and lots of salt and pepper together.
- Add the tofu pieces, stir until completely coated and let sit for 5 minutes.
- Heat the grill on high. Cover the grill tray with a piece of foil (turned up at the edges to catch juices).
- Prepare four equal skewers by threading a piece of onion, tofu, and bell pepper. You should get two sets of onion, tofu, and bell pepper on each skewer.
- Make sure the ingredients aren't squeezed too much.
- The rest of the marinade with yogurt and fresh parsley
- Mix. Gently brush this onto all of the skewers on all sides.
- Place on the prepared grill tray. Place under the hot grill for about 5 minutes until one side is brown, then turn and cook for another 5 minutes, until everything is cooked through and the vegetables are soft and slightly charred.

Fresh Saag Paneer

Preparation time: 10 minutes
Cooking time: 10 minutes
279 calories

Ingredients:

- ✓ 2 teaspoons of rapeseed oil
- ✓ 200 g paneer, cut into cubes
- ✓ Salt and freshly ground black pepper
- ✓ 1 red onion, chopped
- ✓ 1 small thumb (3 cm) fresh ginger, peeled and cut into matches
- ✓ 1 clove of garlic, peeled and thinly sliced
- ✓ 1 green chili, pitted
- ✓ 100 g cherry tomatoes sliced, halved
- ✓ ½ teaspoon ground coriander
- ✓ ½ teaspoon ground cumin
- ✓ ¼ teaspoon ground turmeric
- ✓ ½ teaspoon mild chili powder
- ✓ ½ teaspoon salt
- ✓ 100 g fresh spinach leaves
- ✓ small handful (10 g) parsley, chopped
- ✓ Small handful (10 g) coriander, chopped

Portioning: (2 portions)

Preparation:

- Heat the oil in a pan with a wide lid over high heat. Season the paneer generously with salt and pepper and add to the pan.
- Fry for a few minutes until golden brown, stirring frequently. Remove from pan with a slotted spoon and set aside.
- Reduce the heat and add the onion. Fry for 5 minutes before adding the ginger, garlic and chili.
- Let simmer for a few minutes before adding the cherry tomatoes. Put the lid on the pan and cook for another 5 minutes.
- Add the spices and salt and stir. Place the paneer back in the pan and stir until coated.
- Put the spinach in the pan with the parsley and coriander and put the lid on.
- Let the spinach wilt for 1–2 minutes, then add it to the bowl. Serve immediately.

Fragrant Asian Hotpot

Preparation time: 15 minutes
Cooking time: 10 minutes
185 calories

Ingredients:
- 1 teaspoon tomato paste
- 1 star anise, crushed (or 1 teaspoon ground anise)
- Small handful (10 g) parsley, stalks finely chopped
- Small handful (10 g) coriander, stalks finely chopped
- Juice of 1 lime 500 ml chicken broth,
- ½ carrot, peeled and cut into matches
- 50 g broccoli, cut into small florets
- 50 g sprouts
- 100 g raw tiger prawns
- 100 g firm tofu, chopped
- 50 g rice noodles, cooked according to package instructions
- 50 g boiled water chestnuts, drained
- 20 g sushi ginger, chopped
- 1 tbsp good quality miso paste

Portioning: (2 portions)

Preparation:
- Put the tomato paste, star anise, parsley stalks, coriander stalks, lime juice and chicken in a large pan and simmer for 10 minutes.
- Add the carrots, broccoli, prawns, tofu, noodles and water chestnuts and simmer gently until the prawns are cooked. Remove from the heat and stir in the sushi ginger and miso paste. Serve sprinkled with parsley and coriander leaves.

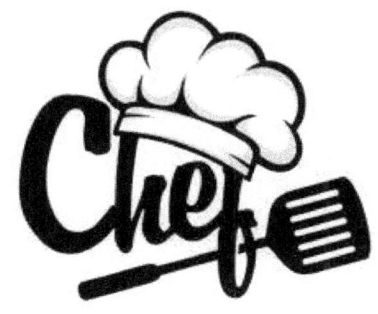

Quick fried beef with salsa verde

Preparation time: 10 minutes
Cooking time: 15 minutes
335 calories

Ingredients:
- ✓ 10 g flat parsley, finely chopped
- ✓ 2 basil leaves, chopped
- ✓ 2 mint leaves, chopped
- ✓ 2 cocktail pickles, finely chopped
- ✓ 1 teaspoon capers, drained
- ✓ 2 anchovy fillets, drained and chopped
- ✓ 1 teaspoon of red wine vinegar juice from 1 lime
- ✓ 1 tsp Dijon mustard
- ✓ 1 teaspoon extra virgin olive oil
- ✓ 100 g broccoli, cut into small florets
- ✓ 2 × 150 g beef schnitzel
- ✓ Salt and freshly ground black pepper

Portioning: (2 portions)

Preparation:
- Put the parsley, basil, mint, pickles, capers, anchovies, vinegar, lime juice, Dijon mustard and extra virgin olive oil in a bowl and stir together.
- Cover and let rest for at least 5 minutes.
- Steam the broccoli over a pan of boiling water for 5 minutes or until just tender.
- Lightly wrap the beef in cling film and beat it with a rolling pin to a thickness of about half a centimeter.
- Remove from the cling film and season with salt and pepper on both sides.
- Heat the rapeseed oil in a pan with a wide lid over high heat. Add the garlic, stir, and immediately add the beef.
- Fry only 1–2 minutes on each side. Turn off the stove, stir in the broccoli, put the lid on the pan and let sit for 3-5 minutes.
- Serve with the drizzled salsa verde.

Teriyaki salmon with Chinese vegetables

Preparation time: 10 minutes
Cooking time: 15 minutes
354 calories

Ingredients:

- ✓ 1 thumb (5 cm) fresh ginger, peeled and grated
- ✓ 1 tbsp soy sauce
- ✓ 1 teaspoon fish sauce
- ✓ 1 teaspoon honey
- ✓ 1 teaspoon sesame oil
- ✓ 2 salmon fillets, skinless, quartered
- ✓ 1 shallot, peeled and thinly sliced
- ✓ ½ carrot, peeled and cut into sticks
- ✓ 1 onion of fennel, thinly sliced
- ✓ 1 onion pak choi, cut
- ✓ 100g kale leaves, stems removed and torn

Portioning: (2 portions)

Preparation:

- In a large bowl, stir together the ginger, soy, fish sauce, honey and sesame oil.
- Place the salmon pieces in the bowl, turn them and cover each piece with the sauce.
- Let it rest while you prepare the rest of the meal. In a large pan with a lid, add about 5 mm - 1 cm of water and bring to the boil.
- Add the shallot, carrot and fennel. Put the lid on the pan and cook for 4 minutes.
- Add the pak choi and kale, stir gently and add a little more water when the pan looks dry. •
- Place the salmon pieces on top of the vegetables and pour in the remaining marinade.

   Put the lid back on the pan and steam for 8 minutes, until the salmon is cooked through.

Kale tomatoes Pasta

Preparation time: 10 minutes
Cooking time: 10 minutes
520 calories

Ingredients:
- ✓ 200 g linguine
- ✓ 200 g cherry tomatoes, halved lemon zest
- ✓ Juice of ½ lemon
- ✓ 50 ml of extra virgin olive oil
- ✓ 1 heaped teaspoon sea salt
- ✓ 500 ml of boiling water
- ✓ 200 g kale leaves, stems removed and roughly torn
- ✓ Large handful (20 g) parsley, finely chopped
- ✓ 20 g parmesan, finely grated
- ✓ Freshly ground black pepper

Portioning: (2 portions)

Preparation:
- Use a large, shallow pan with a lid wide enough to hold the linguine flat. Add the pasta, tomatoes, lemon zest, lemon juice, olive oil and salt to the pan.
- Pour over 500 ml of boiling water, put the lid on and bring it to a boil. Once it boils, remove the lid and stir. Continue to cook and stir every minute for 6 minutes.
- Add the kale and cook for another 2 minutes or until almost all of the water has evaporated.
- Combine the parsley, parmesan and black pepper in a small bowl. Divide the pasta between two bowls and sprinkle the parsley and parmesan mixture on top.

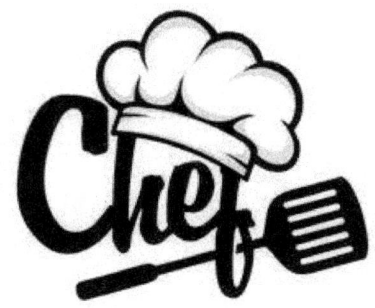

Curry and rice stew

Preparation time: 10 minutes
Cooking time: 15 minutes
347 calories

Ingredients:

- ✓ 2 teaspoons of rapeseed oil
- ✓ 225 g paneer, cut into cubes
- ✓ Salt and freshly ground black pepper
- ✓ 1 red onion, sliced
- ✓ 1 thumb (5 cm) fresh ginger, peeled and grated
- ✓ 2 cloves of garlic, peeled and grated
- ✓ 2 fingers of chili peppers, heads removed and finely chopped
- ✓ ½ teaspoon aniseed
- ✓ 250 g cooked brown rice
- ✓ 250 g ready-to-eat or cooked Puy lentils
- ✓ 100 g frozen soy / edamame beans
- ✓ ½ teaspoon salt
- ✓ ½ teaspoon ground turmeric
- ✓ ½ teaspoon ground cumin
- ✓ ½ teaspoon ground coriander
- ✓ 1 teaspoon mild chili powder
- ✓ 2 tomatoes, chopped
- ✓ 50g baby spinach leaves
- ✓ Large handful (20g) parsley, chopped

Portioning: (2 portions)

Preparation:

- Heat the oil in a large pan over high heat and add the paneer. Season generously with salt and pepper.
- Cook the paneer, stirring frequently, until golden brown all over. Remove with a slotted spoon and set aside.
- Add the onion and reduce the heat in the pan to low. Before adding the ginger, garlic, chili peppers and anise, cook for 2 minutes and cook slowly for another 5 minutes.
- Put the rice and lentils in a large bowl and mix gently, breaking up any lumps and separating the grains.
- If the soybeans are frozen or need to be cooked, cook them according to the directions in the package. Add the salt, ground spices and chili powder to the pan and stir. Add the rice and lentil mixture, soybeans and tomatoes to the pan.
- Stir very well and cook hot. Finally add the spinach and parsley and return the paneer to the pan.
- Stir to combine and serve immediately. After cooling down completely, all spare servings can be chilled and served cold the next day.

Tip to the end

Should you find it difficult to adhere to the recommendation of the very low daily calorie intake.

The increased incorporation of sirtuin-rich foods into a balanced and nutrient-rich menu certainly does no harm and - if not so quickly - in combination with exercise, one or the other pound melts, because the more muscles there are, the more calories are burned.

Practical: Sirtuin-rich foods also inhibit hunger pangs.

Closing words

Sirtfood diet often radicalizes your normal diet by asking you to cut down on meals. While all diets often adhere to some form of calorie limit, it is also important to think about your own lifestyle and think about what you will need throughout the day.

If you're dying to try the sirtfood diet, begin by experimenting by incorporating more of the diet's key staples into what you already eat at home.

Consuming foods rich in polyphenols, including those on the sirtfood list, can help prevent or reduce inflammatory conditions such as cardiovascular disease.

A 2013 study found that diets high in sirtfoods appeared to help with healthy aging and the prevention of chronic diseases.

A 2017 review found that polyphenols appear to help lower body weight, blood sugar and blood pressure.
As you can see, the Sirtuid Diet is a very good way to lose weight in a healthy and, above all, long-term way.

With this in mind, I wish you every success with trying it out and I hope I was able to give you new ideas for a healthier life with this book and the recipes.

CPSIA information can be obtained
at www.ICGtesting.com
Printed in the USA
BVHW051051150221
600147BV00011B/783

9 781801 696333